USING EVIDENCE TO GUIDE
NURSING PRACTICE

D1402314

USING EVIDENCE TO GUIDE
NURSING PRACTICE

2e

Mary Courtney
Helen McCutcheon

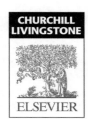

CHURCHILL
LIVINGSTONE

ELSEVIER

Sydney   Edinburgh   London   New York   Philadelphia   St Louis   Toronto

Churchill Livingstone
is an imprint of Elsevier

Elsevier Australia. ACN 001 002 357
(a division of Reed International Books Australia Pty Ltd)
Tower 1, 475 Victoria Avenue, Chatswood, NSW 2067

National Library of Australia Cataloguing-in-Publication Data

Using evidence to guide nursing practice / editors Mary
 Courtney, Helen McCutcheon.

2nd ed.

ISBN: 978 0 7295 3950 0 (pbk.)

Includes index.
Bibliography.

Evidence-based nursing--Australia.
Nursing--Decision making.

McCutcheon, Helen.

610.73

Publisher: Luisa Cecotti
Developmental Editor: Larissa Norrie
Publishing Services Manager: Helena Klijn
Editorial Coordinator: Lauren Allsop
Edited by Alexandra Holliday
Proofread by Maria McGivern
Cover and internal design by Avril Makula
Index by Michael Ferreira
Typeset by TNQ Books & Journals Pvt Ltd
Printed in Australia by Ligare

PEFC
PEFC/21-31-17

The book has been printed on paper certified
by the Programme for the Endorsement of
Forest Certification (PEFC). PEFC is
committed to sustainable forest management
through third party forest certification
of responsibly managed forests.

Contents

Preface

Over the past decade, the Australian healthcare system has come under siege to improve the quality and access of patient care within a context of increasingly limited resources. Greater emphasis is being placed on the need for all health professionals to seek out evidence for best practice and apply it in their everyday work.

Large gaps remain in the amount of robust evidence for much of what nurses do during the course of their daily work. Therefore, the challenge for nurses is to develop and implement well-focused evidence-based nursing interventions to improve the quality of patient care. Evidence-based practice (EBP) is fundamentally about reducing uncertainty in clinical care, in order to achieve efficient and effective service delivery.

In 2005, the first edition of this book provided a guide for both experienced nurses and students of nursing on how to find, appraise and use appropriate evidence in their everyday practice. This theme continues in the second edition, with a greater emphasis on i) how to develop an EBP culture in the workplace that supports clinicians to make healthcare decisions based on finding and using the best available evidence; and ii) how to translate evidence into practice.

The second edition is divided into five parts:

Part one examines what EBP is. It describes the development of the EBP movement and provides an overview of why EBP has spread so rapidly over the past decade. Part one details types of evidence, describes the relationship between clinical questions and research designs to demonstrate evidence, and examines both quantitative and qualitative means of gathering evidence.

Part two focuses on how to develop a workplace culture that supports EBP. It describes important features of a positive evidence-based work culture and outlines how the reader can assess their own work environment. Part two also discusses the development and use of clinical guidelines.

Part three examines how to locate and appraise evidence. It also describes the process of undertaking a systematic review.

Part four focuses on how to evaluate practice by undertaking a clinical audit and program evaluation.

Part five examines how to translate evidence into practice, including a new case study that can be applied to this purpose.

A range of discussion points and case studies are included throughout the book to assist the reader to understand the material provided in the text.

If you find any errors as you read through this book, please let us know. We will acknowledge your good detective work when the book is reprinted. We will also appreciate any feedback you have that might assist in the refinement of subsequent editions of this text.

Finally, many thanks to the contributing authors for providing the expertise and experience required to draw together the material for the complex issues and practices addressed in this book.

Mary Courtney
Helen McCutcheon

Contributors

Editors

Mary Courtney, RN, BAdmin (Accounting), MHP, PhD, FRCNA, AFACHSE, Acting Executive Dean and Professor of Nursing, Faculty of Health, Queensland University of Technology, Brisbane, Queensland

Helen McCutcheon, RN, RM, BA, MPH, PhD, Professor and Head of School of Nursing and Midwifery, University of South Australia, Adelaide, South Australia

Chapter authors

Kate Andre, PhD, MN, BN, FRCNA, Step 2010 Project Leader, Senior Lecturer, School of Nursing and Midwifery, University of South Australia, Adelaide, South Australia

Sally Borbasi, RN, PhD, MRCNA, Professor of Nursing, School of Nursing and Midwifery, Griffith University, Brisbane, Queensland

Anthea Court, MBA, Associate Director, The Joanna Briggs Institute; Field Associate, School of Population Health and Clinical Practice, University of Adelaide, Adelaide, South Australia

Kate Deuter, BAppSc, Grad Cert, Research Assistant, School of Nursing and Midwifery, University of South Australia, Adelaide, South Australia

Adrian Esterman, PhD, MSc, BSc (Hons), DLSHTM, Foundation Chair of Biostatistics and Professor, School of Nursing and Midwifery, University of South Australia, Adelaide, South Australia

John Field, PhD, RN, DNE, BLegSt, FCN, FRCNA, Associate Professor and Director, Research and Higher Degrees, School of Nursing and Midwifery, University of Tasmania, Tasmania

Glenn Gardner, RN, BAppSc (Adv Nursg), MEdSt, PhD, FRCNA, Professor of Clinical Nursing and Director, Centre for Clinical Nursing, Queensland University of Technology and Royal Brisbane and Women's Hospital, Brisbane, Queensland

David Gillham, PhD, MNSt, BN, BSc, RN, Senior Lecturer School of Nursing and Midwifery, University of South Australia, Adelaide, South Australia

Anna Holasek, BA, Dip Ed, Grad Dip Library and Information Management, User Services Librarian, The Queen Elizabeth Hospital Library, Woodville, South Australia

Debra Jackson, PhD, Professor, School of Nursing and Midwifery, College of Health and Science, University of Western Sydney, Sydney, New South Wales

Kelly Lewis, PhD Candidate, RN, CCRN, BN, BHSc (Hons), Grad Dip Nurs Science (Intensive Care), Lecturer, School of Nursing and Midwifery, University of South Australia, Adelaide, South Australia

Craig Lockwood, RN, BN, GradDip, MNSc, Associate Director, The Joanna Briggs Institute, University of Adelaide, Adelaide, South Australia

Elizabeth Manias, PhD, Cert Crit Care, MPharm, BPharm, MNursStud, RN, FRCNA, MPSA, Professor and Associate Head of Research, Faculty of Medicine, Dentistry and Health Sciences, School of Nursing and Social Work, The University of Melbourne, Melbourne, Victoria

Sonya Osborne, RN, MN, BSN, Grad Cert (Periop Nurs), Grad Cert (Higher Ed), MRCNA, MACORN, CNOR, Centaur Fellow, Lecturer and Coordinator, School of Nursing and Midwifery, Faculty of Health, Queensland University of Technology, Brisbane, Queensland

Barbara Parker, RN, BSc (Hons), Grad Cert Ed (Higher Ed), PhD, Bachelor of Nursing Program Director, School of Nursing and Midwifery, University of South Australia, Adelaide, South Australia

Alan Pearson, RN, PhD, FRCNA, FAAG, FRCN, Executive Director, The Joanna Briggs Institute, Professor of Evidence Based Healthcare, The University of Adelaide, Adelaide, South Australia

Claire Rickard, RN, PhD, FRCNA, Professor, School of Nursing and Midwifery, and Lead, Intravascular Device Research Group, Research Centre for Clinical and Community Practice Innovation, Griffith University, Brisbane, Queensland

Colleen Smith, PhD, MEd, BEd, DipAppSc (NEd), RN, Senior Lecturer, School of Nursing and Midwifery, University of South Australia, Adelaide, South Australia

Joy Vickerstaff, MCogSci, BA, RN, RM, DNE, DAN, Grad Cert Hlth Econ, FCN

Jane Warland, Dip Appl Sc (Nurs), RN, RM, PhD, Grad Cert (University Teaching), Lecturer, School of Nursing and Midwifery, University of South Australia, Adelaide, South Australia

Joan Webster, BA, RN, Nursing Director (Research), Royal Brisbane and Women's Hospital; Adjunct Associate Professor, School of Nursing and Midwifery, Queensland University of Technology and University of Queensland; Adjunct Professor, Research Centre for Clinical and Community Practice Innovation, Griffith University, Brisbane, Queensland

Reviewers

Sharon Andrew, PhD, MSc (Hons), BAppSc, RN, RM, FRCNA, Senior Lecturer, Learning and Teaching Fellow, School of Nursing and Midwifery, Faculty of Health and Science, University of Western Sydney, Sydney, New South Wales

Brigid Gillespie, RN, Cert Periop, BHlthSc (Hons), PhD, Lecturer and Research Ethics Adviser, School of Nursing and Midwifery, Griffith University Gold Coast Campus, Gold Coast, Queensland

Ann McKillop, MA, RN, Senior Lecturer, School of Nursing, Faculty of Medical and Health Sciences, The University of Auckland, Auckland, New Zealand

Christine Mercer, PhD, MEd, BA (Soc Sci), RN, FCNANZ, Senior Lecturer, School of Nursing and Health Studies, Waiariki Institute of Technology, Rotorua, New Zealand

PART ONE

Introduction

CHAPTER 1

Evidence-based nursing practice

Mary Courtney, Claire Rickard, Joy Vickerstaff and Anthea Court

1.1 Learning objectives

After reading this chapter, you should be able to:
1. understand what evidence-based practice (EBP) is
2. understand the benefits and alternatives to using EBP
3. explain what has caused the major spread of the EBP movement
4. list where evidence may be located to support best practice
5. describe two major structures promoting the utilisation of EBP in Australia—the National Institute of Clinical Studies (NICS) and the Joanna Briggs Institute (JBI)
6. explain how evidence may be incorporated into nursing practice, and
7. discuss the challenges the EBP-based movement has posed for both nursing education and nursing research.

1.2 Introduction

This chapter introduces the reader to the development of the evidence-based practice (EBP) movement and provides an overview of why EBP has spread so rapidly over the past 15 years. It explains how evidence may be incorporated into nursing practice and examines the challenges the EBP-based movement has posed for both nursing education and nursing research.

1.3 What is 'evidence-based practice'?

Health professionals currently advise their patients to stop smoking. Why do they give this advice? Why don't they advise them to start smoking or increase their smoking intake? The reason is that evidence is available which demonstrates:
- high levels of smoking are associated with increased risk of lung cancer, and
- stopping smoking reduces the risk of lung cancer.

This is an example of evidence that can identify the cause of a disease and the effectiveness of an intervention to improve patient outcomes and decrease illness and disability.

The development of EBP can be traced back to the work of a group of researchers at McMaster University in Ontario, Canada, who set out to redefine the practice of medicine to improve the usability of information (Lockett 1997).

The term 'evidence-based practice', or EBP, has been derived from the earlier work of evidence-based medicine. Earlier years saw the development of EBP limited to the discourse of 'medicine'; however, more recently many other health professional groups have moved to use EBP principles in their practice—for example, orthodontics (Harrison 2000) and allied health therapies (Bury & Mead 1998).

In 1997, Sackett et al (1997:2) published the first textbook on evidence-based medicine and defined it as:

> The conscientious, explicit and judicious use of current best evidence in making decisions about the healthcare of patients.

In 2000, Sackett et al (2000) also included patient values as well as clinical expertise:

> The practice… integrates clinical expertise and patient values with the best available research evidence.

Critics of EBP have described it as 'cookbook' healthcare, or the worship of science above human experience. However, these criticisms are easily defused by an understanding of the three-factor interaction that EBP promotes: the best available research evidence; clinical expertise; and patient values (see Fig 1.1).

The *Journal of the American Medical Association (JAMA)* has been committed to publishing 'Users' guides' to the research literature, with an excellent series of 25 articles on the topic published from 1993 to 2000. An important resource is a compendium of these articles, with further commentary, published in book form in 2002 (Guyatt & Rennie 2002). Although the guides are aimed primarily at a medical audience, they are highly appropriate for all health practitioners, including not only traditional quantitative/epidemiological approaches but also guides to interpreting qualitative evidence for practice (Giacomini & Cook 2000a, 2000b).

Therefore, EBP is not only applying research-based evidence to assist in making decisions about the healthcare of patients, but rather extends to identifying knowledge gaps, and finding, systematically appraising and condensing the evidence to assist clinical expertise, rather than replace it (Elshaug et al 2009).

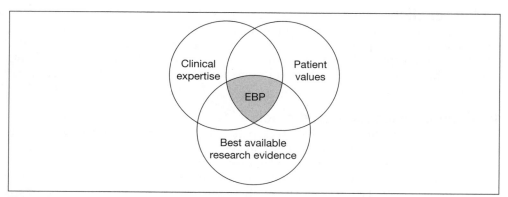

Figure 1.1 The three elements of evidence-based practice
Source: Sackett et al 2000

1.4 **What are the benefits of evidence-based practice?**

There are benefits of EBP for patients/consumers, nurses, healthcare organisations and the community.

1.4.1 **For patients/consumers**

To healthcare consumers, it may seem ludicrous, or even frightening, that the EBP concept is relatively new. Patients typically accept recommended care from health professionals with the unspoken assumption that the practitioner knows what works.

1.4.2 **For nurses**

In an ideal world, nurses could keep up to date by reading all of the published literature in their relevant area. In reality, with approximately a thousand new publications each year relevant just to surgical nursing, for example, this is clearly an impossible task. EBP allows a more structured and streamlined way of keeping abreast of relevant new developments without becoming overwhelmed by information overload.

EBP also allows nurses to communicate effectively with their patients and with the healthcare team about the rationales for decision making and care plans. An EBP nurse is a confident professional, feeling assured that they are providing care which is supported by facts rather than habits, and can take legal accountability for their practice.

1.4.3 **For healthcare organisations**

A commitment to EBP philosophy allows healthcare organisations to position themselves in the market as quality institutions. An EBP-compliant institution should be less likely to attract litigation, and will be able to successfully defend the care delivered if it was in line with international best evidence at the time of care. In addition, EBP allows the scrutinising of practice for effectiveness. This process often results in practice changes that allow significant cost savings, or alternatively justify necessary additional expenditure. This is attractive to organisations frequently struggling to meet assigned budgetary limits, or lobbying government for additional funds.

1.4.4 **For the community**

Through the utilisation of EBP, finite resources are not wasted on the delivery of ineffective interventions. Additionally, EBP limits the amount of disability and suffering throughout the community by ensuring the most current and effective care is provided.

1.5 **What are the alternatives to evidence-based practice?**

You may be wondering how nurses made decisions about their practice before the relatively recent EBP movement, or even what the alternatives to EBP are. If we are honest, for most of our working life we function on 'automatic pilot'; that is, we ritualistically do things the way we have always done them, the way we were taught as a student or graduate nurse, or just in the 'accepted' way of doing things in our current workplace.

However, at times our comfort zone is challenged, and we identify a knowledge deficit when confronting an unusual or challenging problem. At times like these, practitioners may guide their practice by asking the opinion of colleagues or senior practitioners, reviewing employer policies, reading textbooks or lecture notes, leafing through nursing or other journals, and listening to speakers at professional conferences or other education forums. Can you think of some benefits and limitations to these methods of guiding practice? For example, if a decision needs to be made immediately, guidance from an experienced colleague or organisational manual provides a quick and easy reference tool. However, on the downside, even well-meaning and senior practitioners may not have the latest knowledge, and policy manuals are frequently out-of-date, even if they were prepared using the best evidence at the time of policy development.

1.6 Why the rapid spread of evidence-based practice?

Some of the major reasons cited by Sackett et al (1997) for the spread of the EBP movement have been the:

- lack of research-based information to support clinical decision making
- lack of research-based guidelines and protocols to use in clinical practice
- overwhelming volume and variability of new journal information, and
- inadequacy of traditional sources of information (e.g. textbooks out-of-date).

However, health departments around the world are increasingly being stretched to cover ever-rising health expenditures and, with treatment and care costs increasing all the time, governments need to ensure they are using public funds for treatment and care that is effective with positive health outcomes and benefits for the public.

While it may be commendable to take the view that health departments have encouraged the development of EBP because they genuinely wish for patients to receive the best available care and to have the fewest adverse events possible, unfortunately, the reality may more likely be that ineffective care and adverse events are very costly in terms of extended lengths of stay in expensive hospital beds and require additional costs such as pharmaceuticals, pathology tests and radiography. Additionally, poor patient care and mistakes also lead to threats of litigation (Tarling & Crofts 2002).

While EBP was initially limited to the practice of medicine it became clear that unless all the members of the health team embraced EBP it would have limited impact.

1.7 Where is the evidence located?

Evidence for practice decisions is increasingly available in online format. Some resources are available free of charge, while others attract a fee for use, although staff and students of healthcare facilities and universities can usually access these through the institution at no personal cost. Many electronic resources now provide links to full-text journal articles for some records. New products are constantly being developed to allow practitioners to quickly and easily search for relevant evidence. Some of the currently well-established and recommended sources of evidence are described below.

1.7.1 CINAHL®

The CINAHL® (Cumulative Index to Nursing and the Allied Health Literature) database covers the nursing, allied health and health sciences literature from 1982 to the present. Originally a printed index, the CINAHL database has been available as a web-based product since 1994. CINAHL includes 1.7 million records and is growing weekly. Individuals can subscribe to CINAHL for a fee; however, as most health facilities and universities are subscribers, access is available free to their staff and students. Contact your librarian to find out whether your institution has CINAHL access (see www.ebsco host.com/cinahl).

1.7.2 MEDLINE®

MEDLINE® (Medical Literature Analysis and Retrieval System Online) is compiled by the US National Library of Medicine and is acknowledged as the world's most comprehensive source of bibliographic information for health. MEDLINE includes literature from the nursing, medicine and allied health disciplines, as well as the health humanities, and dentistry, veterinary, biological, physical and information science. MEDLINE has more than 17 million records dating from 1965 to the present and is updated weekly. Subscription through various commercial platforms is available for a fee to both individuals and institutions, and is widely available for free to staff and students of subscribing health facilities and universities. MEDLINE is also available free of charge from any computer connected to the internet through a platform called PubMed® (see www.ncbi.nlm.nih.gov/PubMed).

1.7.3 The Cochrane Library

An important resource for EBP is the Cochrane Library, which is produced by the international Cochrane Collaboration. Material included has been prefiltered for quality of evidence and clinical applicability, and is updated quarterly. The Library consists of several databases.

The Cochrane Database of Systematic Reviews (CDSR) was launched in 2000 and includes over 5546 full-text systematic reviews of high-quality research undertaken by Cochrane collaborators that are designed to answer specific clinical questions. The Database of Abstracts of Reviews of Effects (DARE) includes over 9025 structured abstracts of systematic reviews undertaken outside the Cochrane Collaboration. The Cochrane Central Register of Controlled Trials (CENTRAL) includes details of over 550,000 controlled trials published in journals, as well as reports from conference proceedings and other sources not currently listed in other bibliographic databases.

Other materials include the Cochrane Methodology Register (CMR), the National Health Service Economic Evaluation Database (NHSEED) and the Health Technology Assessment (HTA) database. All residents of Australia can access the Cochrane Library for free online due to funding provided by the Commonwealth Government and administered by the National Institute of Clinical Studies (NICS). Follow the link to the Cochrane Library at www.nhmrc.gov.au/nics.

1.7.4 PsycINFO®

The PsycINFO® database is the premier online collection of bibliographic references covering psychological literature from 1872 to the present, including articles from over 1300 journals. Most references include abstracts or content summaries. In addition to journal articles, many books, chapters and academic dissertations are included. PsycINFO is a fee-for-product service that is widely available at no charge to practitioners through subscribing health libraries (see www.apa.org/psycinfo).

1.7.5 Meditext

Meditext was launched in 2001 and contains material from the Australasian Medical Index (AMI) compiled by the National Library of Australia. Indexed are over 150 Australian and New Zealand health journals and other materials such as conference proceedings and government reports. Many Meditext references are materials not included in MEDLINE. Some full-text documents and links to full-text articles are included. The majority of universities and health departments provide fee-free access to their staff and students.

Further discussion on how to locate evidence is provided in Chapter 5, while Chapter 6 provides in-depth coverage on how to locate evidence when undertaking a systematic review.

1.7.6 The Joanna Briggs Institute

The Joanna Briggs Institute (JBI) provides a database of evidence summaries (literature reviews) that review international literature on common healthcare interventions and activities. These summaries are linked to care bundles or procedures that describe and/or recommend practice. A database of systematic reviews, predominantly relevant to nursing and increasingly to allied health, is also located on the JBI website. These resources are available to subscribing members of the Institute. Many Australian healthcare facilities are members of the Institute and therefore provide free access to this information for their staff. Additionally, *Best Practice* information sheets—four-page summaries of results and recommendations for practice based on systematic reviews of research—are accessible free of charge (see www.joannabriggs.edu.au).

1.7.7 The 'grey' literature

The 'grey' literature is a term used to refer to evidence that exists in some format but is difficult to find due to its non-inclusion in searchable bibliographic indexes such as MEDLINE, which predominantly contain references to articles in highly ranked peer-refereed journals. While some grey literature may not be contained in such journals because it is of poor quality, this is not always the case, and a thorough literature search will also make efforts to identify relevant research that may have been published only in conference proceedings, non-refereed journals, government/organisational reports, textbooks or the popular press, as well as academic theses that may not have been followed up with publication. Some efforts have been made to assist clinicians to search or access the grey literature including aspects of the Cochrane Collaboration (see Section 1.7.3) and the following online instruments: the Australasian Digital Theses (ADT) Program and the Conference Papers Index.

1.7.7.1 The Australasian Digital Theses Program

The Australasian Digital Theses (ADT) Program began in 1998 and has been open to all Australian universities since 2000. It consists of a national collaborative of digitised theses produced at Australian universities (PhD and Masters by Research theses only). The program can be accessed free of charge via any internet-connected computer (see www.adt.caul.edu.au).

1.7.7.2 The Conference Papers Index

This database provides over 2.5 million citations to oral papers and poster sessions presented at major scientific conferences internationally from 1982 to the present. Major areas of subject coverage include healthcare, as well as biochemistry, chemistry, biology, biotechnology and many others. The Index is updated bimonthly and is available through subscribing health or academic institutions (see www.csa.com/factsheets/cpi-set-c.php).

1.8 Major structures promoting evidence-based practice

In Australia and New Zealand, the major structures promoting EBP are the National Health and Medical Research Council (NHMRC)'s National Institute of Clinical Studies (NICS), the Joanna Briggs Institute (JBI), and the New Zealand Guidelines Group (NZGG).

1.8.1 The National Institute of Clinical Studies

Reliable data on the gaps between clinical evidence (what research shows that clinicians should be doing in their clinical care) and clinical practice (what is actually done) is often difficult to find. Despite this, there have been sufficient published research studies to suggest that there is a gap problem in many healthcare systems. Dutch and American studies indicate that 30–40% of patients do not receive care based on the best research evidence, and that 20–25% of the care provided is either not needed or may be potentially harmful (Grol 2001, Schuster et al 1998).

The National Institute of Clinical Studies (NICS) is Australia's national agency for improving healthcare by helping to close the gaps between best available evidence and current clinical practice. It was established as an Australian Government-owned company, run by a board of directors directly appointed by the Minister for Health, and commenced operations in 2001. On 1 April 2007, the NICS merged with the NHMRC in order to provide the NHMRC with the capacity to drive implementation of the clinical practice guidelines it develops and endorses (NHMRC 2008). The NICS and the NHMRC are working jointly on several projects, including a revision of the national infection control guidelines. In addition, a guide to the development, implementation and evaluation of clinical practice guidelines is underway.

1.8.1.1 Why the need for the NICS?

In an editorial in the *Medical Journal of Australia* (Silagy 2001), the inaugural Chair of the NICS, the late Chris Silagy, observed that the language and concepts of evidence-based healthcare have become institutionalised in most spheres of healthcare, yet there are still significant gaps between evidence and practice.

Silagy noted that since the inception of evidence-based medicine there has been considerable emphasis on what he termed 'upstream' strategies to support EBP, an emphasis characterised by huge numbers of systematic reviews, health technology assessments and clinical guidelines being made available to clinicians. This emphasis, however, had come without adequate consideration of the 'downstream' strategies necessary to ensure effective uptake and implementation of best evidence by clinicians. The mission of the NICS is to assist clinicians to turn this evidence into action.

1.8.1.2 What is important?

In planning a strategy to address the evidence–practice gaps in Australia, one of the first tasks of the NICS was to work with clinicians in a series of consultation rounds to identify the gaps that are considered widespread, clinically significant and urgent. Professional colleges, societies, special interest groups and policy-making bodies were all invited to make submissions and the views of nurses, who make up over 70% of the Australian healthcare workforce, were particularly sought. The consultation process identified a number of clinical areas, including the care of patients treated in emergency departments and the care of patients with heart failure, as suboptimal when compared to best research evidence.

In 2002, the NICS established a nursing reference group of clinicians and academics to offer high-level advice on important practice gaps, and as a result of their recommendations, the NICS began work to scope opportunities to close the gaps in pain management and pressure-area management. This led to the NICS embarking on a major project to improve pain management in hospitalised patients with cancer, while the latter recommendation led the NICS to scope pressure-area care in Australia (see www.nhmrc.gov.au/nics).

Identification of EBP gaps is an evolutionary process and, in 2003, the NICS published the first in a projected series of reports highlighting important gaps identified by doctors, nurses, allied health clinicians and policy makers in Australia (NICS 2003). In 2005, a review of this report was undertaken (NICS 2005a) to provide a fresh look at what progress had been made in closing the gaps identified in the original report. Additionally, in 2005, a second volume in the series of evidence–practice gap reports was published, highlighting several areas where gaps between evidence and practice remain in day-to-day practice (NICS 2005b). See Appendix 1.1 for further details of clinical topics covered in these reports.

As our understanding of what actually happens in clinical practice improves and we look more deeply through better integration of routine data-collection systems at the surgery and bedside, it is anticipated that many more clinically significant gaps will be identified in the coming years.

1.8.1.3 What do we know about what works?

The second task of the NICS was to bring together the disparate body of work on changing clinician behaviour into a coherent whole. Industries such as mining and aviation have approached behaviour change in a two-pronged way, from both a systemic and an individual perspective. While there is still an emphasis on individual responsibility, there has also been a corresponding reduction in the discretion of individuals to act autonomously, in favour of the introduction of industry-wide systems and protocols. This has resulted in significant improvements in safety. Attempts to change clinical behaviour in the healthcare industry have, to date, focused almost exclusively on the role of the individual clinician in areas such as supporting individual clinical decision making, and there have been very few initiatives that have looked at system-wide approaches to change. One important factor that has inhibited more widespread attempts at system-wide improvement is the lack of a sound scientific evidence base for the many strategies that have been proposed to date.

The NICS also aims to use expertise from areas such as behavioural psychology and marketing to better identify ways of systematically changing clinician behaviour in Australia. In 2003, the NICS convened a national workshop of clinicians and policy makers with an expertise in change management to identify better ways to manage change in Australian healthcare; the results of the workshop were published in 2004 (NICS 2004).

1.8.1.4 Clinical leaders

The third task of the NICS has been to foster clinical champions for change in Australia. In a series of programs that offer targeted grants, fellowships, scholarships and research funding in a variety of settings, the NICS hopes to identify and nurture clinicians in their early-to-mid careers who, supported by the NICS expertise in change management, will become Australia's next generation of clinical leaders.

These leaders face significant barriers. Implementation of research is still the poor relation of primary research and many clinicians face unique pressures as they try to implement change. Potential clinical leaders are often trapped by the competing requirements of teaching and clinical care, particularly in the context of severe workforce shortages, and it is hoped that the fellowship program in particular will allow clinicians 'space' to devote time and energy to developing large-scale implementation programs.

One important role the NICS is taking to support clinical leaders is to lobby research funders in Australia to commit a greater proportion of research grants to studies of the implementation of primary research.

1.8.1.5 Working with others

The fourth task of the NICS is to develop tools to assist clinicians in implementing evidence-based healthcare. In 2002, the NICS acted on behalf of the Australian Government to purchase open access to the Cochrane Library, the best available source of appraised clinical evidence on the effects of intervention, for all Australian residents. Recognising the difficulty many clinicians and consumers face in navigating the library's interface, the NICS has worked with the Australasian Cochrane Centre to produce a comprehensive online users' guide to the library (see www.cochrane.org.au/libraryguide).

Other tools developed by the NICS for clinicians include a range of literature reviews on diverse topics such as factors supporting high performance in healthcare organisations and the effectiveness of clinical information services (see Appendix 1.1); a scanning service where relevant journals and websites are regularly monitored; a database linking Australian-based clinical effectiveness researchers; and the development of sophisticated web-based tools to support collaborative projects.

The NICS works closely with colleges, societies and organisations representing primary care, hospital medicine, nursing, allied health and indigenous health, as well as national and state-based organisations working in the areas of quality and safety, rural and remote care, guideline development and health insurance. It is only through close relationships with clinicians and policy makers at the clinical interface that the NICS is able to help close EBP gaps. The NICS will continue to build strong working alliances with both Australian and international organisations to improve healthcare.

Australia is not alone in recognising and addressing EBP gaps; strong relationships have been built with groups in New Zealand, Sweden, the UK, Canada, the USA and the Netherlands. The NICS has embarked on a long-term program inviting overseas experts to Australia to share their experiences and foster international dialogue on common problems. Despite workforce challenges and EBP gaps, most of the healthcare delivered in Australia is of a very high standard, and the NICS has a role both in sharing Australian solutions and seeking answers to local problems.

1.8.1.6 The future
Nursing remains a crucial area of engagement for the NICS. As the numerically largest discipline that delivers most of the direct clinical care throughout all sectors of Australian healthcare, nurses are critical to the success of strategies to effectively close the gaps between evidence and practice. Nurses have been instrumental to the success of the work of the NICS in emergency care and will be central to the NICS strategy to improve the assessment and management of pain in hospitalised cancer patients. As the work of the NICS now moves into primary care and chronic disease management, it is ever-more important to identify, understand and disseminate nursing solutions throughout the Australian healthcare system.

1.8.2 The Joanna Briggs Institute
The JBI was established in 1996 as the Joanna Briggs Institute for Evidence-Based Nursing. The Institute has since expanded to include many disciplines and brings together a range of practice-oriented research activities to increase the effectiveness of healthcare practice and improvement of healthcare outcomes by:
- synthesising evidence (through systematic reviews of quantitative and qualitative research)
- transferring evidence (through education and both hard copy and electronic publications), and
- utilising evidence (through implementation projects and evaluation).

Central to the operations of the Institute is the importance of working with healthcare providers, and the belief that research direction should be derived from the current information needs of practice (global health) and result in improved health outcomes (Jordan et al 2006, Pearson et al 2005).

From its very small beginnings in 1996, the JBI is now a growing, dynamic international collaboration of over 500 researchers across 31 countries.

1.8.2.1 The Joanna Briggs Collaboration
The Joanna Briggs Collaboration (see www.joannabriggs.edu.au/about/home.php) is a coordinated effort by a group of self-governing collaborative centres, coordinated through

the leadership of the JBI. The operations of the Joanna Briggs Collaboration include: the conduct of systematic reviews; the development of *Best Practice* information sheets; the promotion of evidence-based healthcare; education and training; the implementation of EBP; and the conduct of evaluation cycles and primary research arising out of systematic reviews.

Collaborating centres are partners supported by academic institutions and/or healthcare facilities that accept the terms of the JBI Memorandum of Understanding. Centres receive modest funding from the Institute each year, but are expected to seek funds within their jurisdiction. Some centres have a geographic jurisdiction, while others have a specialist jurisdiction. The Joanna Briggs Collaboration currently consists of 55 collaborating centres and groups across the world. See Appendix 1.2 for a comprehensive list of collaborators.

1.8.2.2 Membership

In 1996, the first chair of the JBI management committee, Associate Professor Kaye Challinger, predicted that the new institute would have a positive influence on nursing and healthcare delivery. Now, the JBI and its membership fees from the broad membership base, consisting primarily of healthcare and education facilities, financially supports research conducted by the JBI. Institute members receive access to a variety of evidence-based information to inform clinical practice, such as journals and other publications of the JBI, as well as online resources and frameworks to assist with the implementation of evidence and evaluation of outcomes.

The JBI website (see www.joannabriggs.edu.au) has also proven to be a useful tool for both students and practising health professionals. To provide access to the best available evidence to as many practising health professionals as possible, a number of the JBI's resources are available on the website at no cost. Much of the information produced by the JBI is available both electronically and in hard copy to improve accessibility to a wide range of users. Despite the lower cost of providing electronic information, the Institute recognises the continued need for producing hard copy materials for healthcare professionals with limited or no internet access. The Institute works with interested groups in developing countries to provide information and trains local researchers to generate information of most relevance to them.

1.8.2.3 Institute activities

One of the core activities of the JBI is to synthesise and transfer research information relevant to clinical practice. As many nursing questions are not limited to effectiveness, the Institute has used emerging systematic review methodology and developed software to assist in the conduct of comprehensive systematic reviews. SUMARi (System for the Unified Management, Assessment and Review of Information) has been developed to provide researchers with an online system that facilitates the conducting of systematic reviews which consider a variety of research on a specific topic, including qualitative, narrative and opinion, economic data as well as quantitative papers. The inclusion of these research types is most appropriate for healthcare issues that cannot be measured by way of randomised controlled trial. The inclusion of qualitative research has also led to the consideration of the Feasibility, Appropriateness and Meaningfulness of an intervention as well as simply the Effectiveness (i.e. the JBI-initiated FAME scale [Pearson 2004]). This is discussed further in Chapter 6.

Based on the results of systematic reviews, the Institute develops *Best Practice* information sheets, a series designed specifically to provide health professionals with the best available evidence to inform care delivery. Unlike traditional guidelines, the information sheets are not developed for a specific context but present the best available international research evidence on a given topic to inform practice, with the expectation that health professionals will use this evidence together with their clinical judgement and due consideration of their client's preference and the context in which they are providing care. As a reminder of this, each information sheet now includes the JBI 'pebble' of evidence-based practice (Pearson et al 2005). The first *Best Practice* information sheet was produced in September 1997 and distributed through nursing journals in Australia and New Zealand. Dissemination of these information sheets is now global, with copies being freely available on the Institute website, appearing in nursing journals across the world, and being translated into languages other than English including Italian, Spanish, Japanese, Thai and Romanian, with further translation in progress with China.

One of the challenges continuing to face researchers who produce guidelines in the twenty-first century is that of utilisation. It has been recognised for some time that distributing evidence-based guidelines alone does not alter clinical practice and that change management strategies need to be employed to achieve and maintain valuable change (NHS Centre for Reviews and Dissemination 1999). To assist with this critical process, researchers at the JBI have developed and continue to improve the Practical Application of Clinical Evidence System (PACES) tool. PACES is designed to assist healthcare facilities to audit practice using evidence-based audit criteria. This program incorporates the GRIP (Getting Research Into Practice) initiative to assist in the identification and examination of resources and barriers, and facilitate the design of a change plan that may then be followed by a second audit and comparison of outcomes between audits.

Evaluating the influence of the JBI-produced information on healthcare delivery is necessary to determine the benefit of continuing research of this type. Previously the impact of the *Best Practice* series along with its recommendations was evaluated by way of surveys conducted throughout Australia and New Zealand. Survey results indicated that of those who had read *Best Practice*, around 25% of first-survey respondents specifically altered their practice. This figure increased to over 35% in the second survey just 3 years later. Currently, 'before-and-after'-style multisite evaluations are also being conducted to examine the effect of recommendations of *Best Practice* in the clinical setting using PACES.

Critical appraisal skills are also promoted and supported by the JBI. RAPid (Rapid Appraisal Protocol internet database) has been developed as a training program to organise, conduct and archive an evidence summary of the findings of a single study or systematic review. RAPid facilitates study-type recognition, data extraction and the construction of a final report, which may then be submitted online to the RAPid library for independent critique. If it is accepted, it is uploaded for worldwide access. This program is uniquely suitable for use by university lecturers and facilitators of continuing education in health services for training and integration into curricula. RAPid may motivate students to become active in the publication of their work and to experience the benefits of disseminating knowledge to their profession.

It is anticipated that the resources and services of the JBI will continue to develop and grow according to the changing needs of the healthcare profession. The staff of the JBI are committed to regularly examining the resources and services offered. They value user feedback and further develop and improve resources based on this information.

1.8.3 The New Zealand Guidelines Group

The New Zealand Guidelines Group (NZGG) was established in 1996 by the National Health Committee (NHC) as an informal expert network on practice guideline development and implementation. Since 1999, the NZGG has been an independent government-funded society with offices in Wellington and Auckland. Representatives

CASE STUDY: Should central venous line catheter administration sets be changed regularly or left intact?

Modern healthcare involves many invasive procedures and an older, sicker patient population. Unfortunately, procedures may lead to hospital-acquired infections, which significantly increase patient suffering and risk of death, as well as healthcare costs. The most serious form of nosocomial infection is catheter-related bloodstream infection (CRBSI), which involves an infection of the bloodstream secondary to the use of an intravascular catheter.

Nurses are the primary carers of intravascular catheters, and use many strategies in an attempt to prevent CRBSI. Increasingly, these nursing interventions are being subjected to rigorous testing in an attempt to differentiate EBP from historically based practice. Since 1970, nurses have routinely discarded the administration sets attached to intravenous catheters at regular time intervals, and then replaced them with new sets, in the belief that this may reduce the infection risk. Although several studies showed that infection levels did not differ when the administration sets were replaced at different time intervals, no study had ever been undertaken that measured the value of the practice itself.

A randomised controlled trial assigned patients to either have their catheter administration sets replaced routinely, or to have them left intact. It found no statistically significant difference in infection indicators. The study population comprised high-risk intensive-care patients with short-term (7–10 days) central venous catheters. The results of this study provided Level 1A evidence that the expensive and time-consuming procedure of routine administration set replacement is not effective (Rickard et al 2004).

from nursing, Maori Health, Pacific Health, consumer representation, medicine, disability support, public health medicine and general practice govern the NZGG. The role of the NZGG is to provide tools to promote an evidence-based culture within the New Zealand health and disability sector. Activities include production of evidence-based guidelines, distribution of evidence-based information from New Zealand and overseas, and training in guideline development and implementation (see www.nzgg.org.nz).

1.9 How can evidence be incorporated into nursing practice?

There are a variety of situations in which nursing practice and, therefore, nurses draw on the evidence base. Nurses are not only limited to the medical science evidence, but also extend their EBP to the behavioural and social sciences. Some examples are outlined below.

1.9.1 Nursing care intervention evidence

Nurses make clinical decisions about interventions concerning investigations, observations and treatments, and therefore draw upon evidence from a range of different sources. For example, psychosocial evidence as well as pharmacological knowledge may be sought before instigating a particular nursing intervention, as may evidence on cost-effectiveness. Therefore, it is crucial that nurses understand the variety of perspectives of evidence when undertaking an intervention.

1.9.2 Health-related behaviour evidence

Chronic disease is reaching near-epidemic proportions in the developed world. For example, type 2 diabetes is the fastest growing chronic disease of all, and is rapidly becoming a major health issue for ageing populations due to complications such as blindness, loss of limbs and kidney failure. Most complications are preventable if diabetes is self-managed effectively. However, adequate self-management can be difficult to achieve and maintain for many people because of long-established patterns of health behaviour.

To be effective in improving self-management, nurses working with patients with type 2 diabetes need to understand the role that diabetes plays in people's lives, and why it is that some people continue not to follow their planned diet and undertake regular blood glucose checks, even though they are aware of the possible risks of complications.

1.9.3 Models of nursing care delivery evidence

Since nursing comprises the largest proportion of personnel in the provision of healthcare services, satisfaction with nursing care has been found to be the most important predictor of overall satisfaction with hospital care (Abramowitz et al 1987). Research into the determinants of patient satisfaction with nursing care has been conducted from a variety of perspectives, such as outcome of care and nursing care delivery models (Courtney & Wu 2000). There is a wide evidence base within the management sciences on which nurses may draw to explore issues of quality and organisational design.

1.9.4 Management practice evidence

Historic changes are occurring in the healthcare industry. The National Health and Hospitals Reform Commission commissioned the Australian Institute of Health and Welfare (AIHW) to undertake projections of Australian healthcare expenditure for the period 2003–2033 and found total expenditure on health and residential aged care is projected to increase from 9.3% of GDP in 2003–2004 to 12.4% of GDP in 2032–2033 (AIHW 2008). Programs of managed care, expanding outpatient services and day surgery, cost containment, and demands for efficiency and quality outcomes, are transforming the roles of healthcare providers. These changes have meant that nursing executives have had to acquire new skills and competencies to develop a corporate focus. Again, nurses are drawn to the wide management science evidence base in order that they may prepare themselves for the changing roles within their organisations.

1.9.5 Cross-cultural evidence

Nursing care goes far beyond providing a set of treatment interventions. People's experiences, beliefs, attitudes and customs regarding a certain disease or condition can form a stereotype through which physical and emotional sensations may be perceived and interpreted. For example, there is convincing evidence to suggest that menopause is experienced differently by many different ethnic groups (Fu et al 2003). For nurses and other health professionals to provide high-quality care to women undergoing menopause, it is important to look to a range of different evidences. Not only is evidence drawn from medicine, but it is also found in the fields of psychology and sociology, as well as exercise physiology.

The combined results of appropriately appraised international research evidence (see Chs 5 & 6) has value to inform care delivery regardless of the culture in which care is delivered, with the expectation that best available evidence is used along with clinical expertise, consideration of patient values (Sackett et al 2000) and consideration of the context of care (Pearson et al 2005). In different settings and environments, available resources and/or comorbidities may impact on the relevance of certain evidence. For example, research relating to sponging for the treatment of fever in children based in humid climates may not be transferable to the same treatment in temperate climates (Watts et al 2001).

1.10 What is the state of evidence?

EBP is undertaken to support the decisions of nurses and other health professionals to avoid the use of not only ineffective, inappropriate and dangerous treatments, but also treatments that have the potential to be unnecessarily costly. Conversely, EBP is undertaken to identify safe, effective and cost-appropriate care. The four-step process through which EBP may be undertaken is described below and is used as an overarching framework for this book.

1.10.1 Step 1: Developing a workplace culture that supports evidence-based practice

It is important to develop a workplace culture that supports clinicians to make healthcare decisions based upon finding and using the best available evidence, and combining this with their clinical expertise, knowledge and skill, as well as their knowledge of the patient. Chapter 3 describes important features of a positive evidence-based work culture and how to assess your own organisation in relation to these features. Chapter 3 also suggests a range of strategies for developing and sustaining an EBP culture that may work in your organisation. The development and use of evidence-based guidelines is examined in further detail in Chapter 4.

1.10.2 Step 2: Finding the evidence—how to locate and appraise current best evidence

Within an evidence-based workplace culture, it is important to understand what current best evidence is available to inform practice and how to find it. However, in order to find the evidence, first it is essential to know what types of questions to ask. Chapter 2 introduces the Patient Intervention Comparison Outcome (PICO) framework on how to generate research questions and also overviews a range of both qualitative and quantitative research designs used in studies to answer such questions. Chapter 2 examines why different research designs are used and how they contribute to providing evidence of best practice.

Armed with the right questions and knowledge of the research designs, a comprehensive literature review is undertaken to identify evidence for best practice, and, if it is not there, gaps in evidence. Chapter 5 provides a case study to examine how to generate research questions (using the PICO framework), and how to locate and appraise evidence. Chapter 6 follows with an in-depth step-by-step guide to undertaking a systematic review of the literature.

1.10.3 Step 3: Evaluating evidence in practice—how to critically evaluate nursing practice

Undertaking a clinical audit or a program evaluation provides an excellent opportunity to evaluate the effect of a nursing intervention on clinical practice and/or patients; this is an essential feature of an evidence-based workplace culture. Chapters 7 and 8 provide details on each of these evaluation tools, respectively.

1.10.4 Step 4: Translating evidence into practice—how to implement evidence in practice

Care pathways are one example of a clinical tool that, when developed from the best available evidence, can improve clinical effectiveness and efficiency. Chapter 9 is a capstone chapter that showcases an approach clinicians and students may use to obtain evidence to justify the need for a more extensive EBP process. A discussion of clinical pathways is provided and the EBP approach is situated within a framework of critical reflection guided by a series of reflective questions. A case study is used to highlight how the approach can be used to examine a clinical question arising from practice. The case study uses a component of a care pathway for a client presenting for an elective total hip replacement and concludes with a scenario-based activity that can be used to apply what you have learned.

1.11 What are the challenges for nursing education and research?

1.11.1 Challenges for nursing research

Over the past 15 years, the Australian healthcare system has increasingly come under siege to improve the quality and access of patient care within a context of increasingly limited resources. Greater emphasis is being placed on all health professionals to seek out best practice evidence and apply it in their everyday practice.

As there are large gaps in the amount of robust evidence for much of what nurses do during the course of their daily work, the challenge for nurses is to develop, trial, evaluate and implement well-focused evidence-based nursing interventions and treatments to improve the quality of patient care.

1.11.2 Challenges for nursing education

Academic schools of nursing are charged with the responsibility of ensuring nursing graduates are adequately prepared to deliver best practice. In addition, graduates need to have instilled an interest and belief that generating evidence (i.e. 'doing' research) is a part of their future professional career. Although undergraduate nursing education has been present within universities in Australia for over 25 years, some may question the extent to which an evidence-based culture is embedded within curricula. Indeed, nursing registration authorities require that current best practice for nursing interventions and treatments be included in curricula and that research methods be undertaken.

However, a major challenge for academics is actually teaching EBP throughout a curriculum rather than teaching one stand-alone unit of EBP content. In order to ensure that students are immersed in an evidence-based culture, content on the manner through which evidence may be found, appraised and used in practice should be incorporated very early in a curriculum and then interwoven throughout every unit of study in the full 3 years of the course.

1.12 DISCUSSION QUESTIONS

1. How do you define evidence-based nursing?
2. Why do nurses need good evidence for clinical practice?
3 Where and how can nurses find quality evidence to inform their practice?
4. Briefly list 10 commonly used nursing interventions/procedures/protocols used during the course of your everyday practice. Describe what types of evidence these are based upon (i.e. research study, textbook, experience or opinion).

1.13 **References**

Abramowitz S, Coté A A, Berry E 1987 Analysing patient satisfaction: a multi analytic approach. *Quality Research Bulletin* 13(4):122–30.

Australasian Digital Theses Program. Available: www.adt.caul.edu.au 23 Apr 2009.

Australian Institute of Health and Welfare 2008 *Projection of Australian health care expenditure by disease, 2003 to 2033.* AIHW, Canberra.

Bury, T J, Mead, J M (eds) 1998 *Evidence-based healthcare: a practical guide for therapists.* Butterworth-Heinemann, Oxford.

CINAHL. Available: www.ebscohost.com/cinahl 23 Apr 2009.

Cochrane Library. Available: www.nhmrc.gov.au/nics 23 Apr 2009.

Cochrane Library. ACC guide to the Cochrane Library. Available: www.cochrane.org.au/libraryguide 23 Apr 2009.

Conference Papers Index. Available: www.csa.com/factsheets/cpi-set-c.php 23 Apr 2009.

Courtney M, Wu M-L 2000 Models of nursing care: a comparative study of patient satisfaction on two orthopaedic wards in Brisbane. *Australian Journal of Advanced Nursing* 17(4):29–34.

Elshaug A, Moss J, Littlejohns P et al 2009 Identifying existing health care services that do not provide value for money. *Medical Journal of Australia* 190(5):269–73.

Fu S-Y, Anderson D, Courtney M 2003 Cross-cultural menopausal experience: comparison of Australian and Taiwanese women. *Nursing and Health Sciences* 5(1):77–84.

Giacomini M K, Cook D J 2000a Users' guide to the medical literature, XXII: qualitative research in health care. Are the results of the study valid? Evidence Based Medicine Working Group. *Journal of the American Medical Association* 284(3):357–62.

Giacomini M K, Cook D J 2000b Users' guide to the medical literature, XXII: qualitative research in health care. What are the results and how do they help me care for my patients? Evidence Based Medicine Working Group. *Journal of the American Medical Association* 284(4):478–82.

Grol R 2001 Successes and failures in the implementation of evidence-based guidelines for clinical practice. *Medical Care* 39(8 Suppl 20):1146–54.

Guyatt G, Rennie D (eds) 2002 *Users' guides to the medical literature: essentials of evidence-based practice.* Evidence Based Medicine Working Group, American Medical Association Press, Chicago, IL.

Harrison J E 2000 Evidence-based orthodontics: how do I assess the evidence? *Journal of Orthodontics* 27(2):189–97.

Joanna Briggs Collaboration. Available: www.joannabriggs.edu.au/about/home.php 23 Apr 2009.

Joanna Briggs Institute. Available: www.joannabriggs.edu.au 23 Apr 2009.

Jordan Z, Donnelly P, Pittman E 2006 *A short history of a BIG idea: the Joanna Briggs Institute 1996–2006.* Ausmed Publications, Melbourne.

Lockett T 1997 Traces of evidence. *Healthcare Today* July/August:16.

MEDLINE. Available: www.ncbi.nlm.nih.gov/PubMed 23 Apr 2009.

National Health Service (NHS) Centre for Reviews and Dissemination 1999 Getting evidence into practice. *Effective Healthcare* 5(1):1–6.

National Institute of Clinical Studies (NICS) 2003 *Evidence–practice gaps report vol. 1.* NICS, Melbourne.

National Institute of Clinical Studies (NICS) 2004 Adopting best evidence in practice. *Medical Journal of Australia* 180(6):s41–2.

National Institute of Clinical Studies (NICS). Available: www.nhmrc.gov.au/nics 23 Apr 2009.

National Institute of Clinical Studies (NICS) 2005a *Evidence–practice gaps report vol. 1: A review of developments 2004–2007.* NHMRC, Commonwealth of Australia, Canberra.

National Institute of Clinical Studies (NICS) 2005b *Evidence–practice gaps report vol. 2.* NHMRC, Commonwealth of Australia, Canberra.

National Health and Medical Research Council (NHMRC) 2008 *Annual report 2008.* NHMRC, Commonwealth of Australia, Canberra.

New Zealand Guidelines Group. Available: www.nzgg.org.nz 23 Apr 2009.

Pearson A, Wiechula R, Court A et al 2005 The JBI model of evidence-based healthcare. *International Journal of Evidence-Based Healthcare* 3(8):207–15.

Pearson A 2004 Balancing the evidence: incorporating the synthesis of qualitative data into systematic reviews. *JBI Reports* 2(2):45–64.

PsycINFO. Available: www.apa.org/psycinfo 23 Apr 2009.

Rickard C, Lipman J, Courtney M et al 2004 Routine changing of intravascular administration-sets does not reduce colonization or infection in central venous catheters. *Infection Control and Hospital Epidemiology* 25(8):650–5.

Sackett D L, Straus S E, Richardson W S et al 1997 *Evidence based medicine: how to practice and teach EBM, 1st edn*. Churchill Livingstone, London.

Sackett D L, Straus S E, Richardson W S et al 2000 *Evidence based medicine: how to practice and teach EBM, 2nd edn*. Churchill Livingstone, London.

Schuster M, McGlynn E, Brook R H 1998 How good is the quality of healthcare in the United States? *Milbank Quarterly* 76(4):517–63.

Silagy C 2001 Evidence-based healthcare 10 years on: is the National Institute of Clinical Studies the answer? (editorial). *Medical Journal of Australia* 175(3):124–5.

Tarling M, Crofts L 2002 *The essential researcher's handbook for nurses and healthcare professionals, 2nd edn*. Bailliere Tindall, London.

Watts R, Robertson J, Thomas G et al 2001 *The nursing management of fever in children*. The Joanna Briggs Institute, Adelaide.

National Institute of Clinical Studies (NICS): Resources available (see www.nhmrc.gov.au/nics)

Evidence–Practice Gaps Report Volume 1: A review of developments 2004–2007 (NICS 2005a)

- Advising on smoking cessation
- Advising on smoking cessation in pregnancy
- Screening for lung cancer with chest X-rays
- Preventing stroke in patients with atrial fibrillation
- Using ACE inhibitor and beta-blocker therapies in heart failure
- Measuring glycated haemoglobin in diabetes management
- Prescribing antibiotics for upper respiratory tract infections and acute bronchitis
- Preventing venous thromboembolism in hospitalised patients
- Preparing for elective colorectal surgery
- Using colonoscopy in colorectal cancer surgery follow-up
- Managing acute and cancer pain in hospitalised patients

Evidence–Practice Gaps Report Volume 2 (NICS 2005b)

- Folic acid supplements
- Promoting and supporting breast feeding
- Reducing the risk of sudden infant death syndrome
- Promoting use of preventers in chronic asthma
- Managing acute mild asthma in the emergency department
- Recognising and managing panic disorder and agoraphobia
- Vaccinating against influenza
- Haemodialysis vascular access
- Achieving blood pressure control
- Optimising care for stroke patients
- Preventing osteoporosis-related fractures reoccurring
- Compression therapy for venous leg ulcers

Literature reviews

- Factors supporting high performance in healthcare organisations
- Institutional approaches to pain assessment and management
- Interventions to improve uptake of venous thromboembolism prophylaxis in hospitals
- The impact of the internet on consumer health behaviour

Emergency Care Evidence in Practice brochures

- Lumbar imaging in acute non-specific low back pain
- Pain medication for acute abdominal pain
- Rate or rhythm control for recurrent atrial fibrillation
- Cervical spine X-rays in trauma
- Management of acute migraine
- Use of ipratropium bromide for acute asthma

Joanna Briggs Institute Collaboration

At the time of writing, the Joanna Briggs Institute (JBI) collaborates with 55 entities.

Collaborating centres are supported by their university and/or healthcare facility to work closely with the Institute by conducting and contributing to research output, promoting evidence-based healthcare and being involved with the strategic planning of the Joanna Briggs Collaboration. Directors of collaborating centres meet by teleconference quarterly and face-to-face annually, providing valuable international networking.

Evidence synthesis groups are self-governing, self-funding collaborators made up of three or more researchers who conduct systematic reviews using the Institute's framework, peer-review and publication processes.

Evidence utilisation groups are self-governing, self-funding collaborators made up of three or more clinicians, quality managers or other personnel committed to the conduct of clinical improvement projects based on the best available evidence.

Australasia

- New South Wales Centre for Evidence-Based Health Care: a collaborating centre of the Joanna Briggs Institute, University of Western Sydney, New South Wales, Australia
- Australian Centre for Evidence-Based Nutrition and Dietetics: a collaborating centre of the Joanna Briggs Institute, University of Newcastle, New South Wales, Australia
- Western Australian Centre for Evidence-Based Nursing and Midwifery: a collaborating centre of the Joanna Briggs Institute, Curtin University of Technology, Perth, Western Australia, Australia
- Dementia Collaborative Research Centre – Consumers, Carers and Social Research, Queensland University of Technology, Queensland, Australia
- Centre for Allied Health Evidence: a collaborating centre of the Joanna Briggs Institute, University of South Australia, South Australia, Australia
- Centre for Evidence-Based Nursing South Australia: a collaborating centre of the Joanna Briggs Institute, Royal Adelaide Hospital and University of Adelaide, South Australia, Australia
- National Evidence-Based Aged Care Unit: a collaborating centre of the Joanna Briggs Institute, Royal Adelaide Hospital and University of Adelaide, South Australia, Australia

- Royal Adelaide Hospital Multidisciplinary Quality Improvement JBI Evidence Utilisation Group, Royal Adelaide Hospital, South Australia, Australia
- Queensland Centre for Evidence-Based Nursing and Midwifery: a collaborating centre of the Joanna Briggs Institute, Mater Health Services, South Brisbane, Queensland, Australia
- Australian Centre for Evidence-Based Community Care: a collaborating centre of the Joanna Briggs Institute, University of Queensland/Blue Care Research and Practice Development Centre, Toowong, Queensland, Australia
- Australian Centre for Rural and Remote Evidence-Based Practice: a collaborating centre of the Joanna Briggs Institute, Toowoomba Health Service District, Toowoomba, Queensland, Australia
- Austin Health JBI Evidence Utilisation Group, Austin Health, Victoria, Australia
- Royal Perth Hospital JBI Evidence Utilisation Group, Royal Perth Hospital, Western Australia, Australia
- Royal Perth Hospital JBI Evidence Synthesis Group, Royal Perth Hospital, Western Australia, Australia
- Centre for Evidence-Based Healthcare Aotearoa: a collaborating centre of the Joanna Briggs Institute, University of Auckland and Auckland District Health Board, Auckland, New Zealand
- Victoria University Wellington Health Evidence Synthesis Group, Victoria University of Wellington, New Zealand

Africa

- University of Botswana JBI Evidence Synthesis Group, University of Botswana, Gaborone, Botswana
- Joanna Briggs Institute Evidence Synthesis Group, Cameroon, Yaoundé, Cameroon
- Joanna Briggs Institute Evidence Synthesis Group, Ethiopia, Jimma University, Jimma, Ethiopia
- Joanna Briggs Institute Evidence Synthesis Group, Kintampo, Kintampo Health Research Centre, Kintampo, Ghana
- Joanna Briggs Institute Evidence Synthesis Group, Kenya, Kenya Medical Research Institute (KEMRI) Centre for Geographic Medicine Research – Coast, Kilifi, Kenya
- Joanna Briggs Institute Evidence Synthesis Group, Malawi, Malaria Alert Centre, College of Medicine, Chichiri Blantyre, Malawi
- Joanna Briggs Institute Evidence Synthesis Group, Nigeria, Dugbe Ibadan, Oyo State, Nigeria
- Joanna Briggs Institute Evidence Synthesis Group, Nigerian Team, University College Hospital, Ibadan, Nigeria
- Joanna Briggs Institute Evidence Synthesis Group, Rwanda, Kigali, Rwanda
- Centre for Evidence Translation, JBI Evidence Synthesis Group, Stellenbosch University, Stellenbosch, South Africa
- South African Centre for Evidence-Based Nursing and Midwifery: a collaborating centre of the Joanna Briggs Institute, University of KwaZulu-Natal, Durban, South Africa
- Joanna Briggs Institute Evidence Synthesis Group, Swaziland HIV, University of Swaziland, Swaziland
- Joanna Briggs Institute Evidence Synthesis Group, Swaziland Maternal, University of Swaziland, Swaziland

- Joanna Briggs Institute Evidence Synthesis Group, Tanzania, National Institute for Medical Research, Dar es Salaam, Tanzania
- Joanna Briggs Institute Evidence Synthesis Group, Uganda, Kampala, Uganda
- Joanna Briggs Institute Evidence Synthesis Group, Zimbabwe, Harare, Zimbabwe

Americas

- Queen's Joanna Briggs Collaboration: a collaborating centre of the Joanna Briggs Institute, Queen's University, Kingston, Ontario, Canada
- Saint Elizabeth Health Care JBI Evidence Synthesis Group, Saint Elizabeth Health Care, Ontario, Canada
- Indiana Center for Evidence-Based Nursing Practice: a collaborating centre of the Joanna Briggs Institute, Purdue University Calumet, School of Nursing, Hammond, Indiana, USA
- New Jersey Center for Evidence-Based Nursing: a collaborating centre of the Joanna Briggs Institute, University of Medicine and Dentistry of New Jersey School of Nursing, Newark, New Jersey, USA
- Evidence-Based Practice Center of Oklahoma: a collaborating centre of the Joanna Briggs Institute, University of Oklahoma, Oklahoma City, Oklahoma, USA

Asia

- Hong Kong Centre for Evidence-Based Nursing: a collaborating centre of the Joanna Briggs Institute, Chinese University of Hong Kong, Hong Kong
- National and Gulf Centre for Evidence-Based Medicine: a collaborating centre of the Joanna Briggs Institute, Riyadh, Kingdom of Saudi Arabia
- Yonsei Evidence-Based Nursing Centre of Korea: a collaborating centre of the Joanna Briggs Institute, Yonsei University College of Nursing, Seoul, Korea
- Yangon Centre for Evidence-Based Health Care: a collaborating centre of the Joanna Briggs Institute, Military Institute of Nursing and Paramedical Science, Yangon, Myanmar
- Fudan Evidence-Based Nursing Centre: a collaborating centre of the Joanna Briggs Institute, Shanghai, People's Republic of China
- Center for Research on Movement Science, University of Santo Tomas, JBI Evidence Synthesis Group, University of Santo Tomas, España, Manila, Philippines
- National Healthcare Group Health Science Outcome Research Collaborating Centre for Evidence-Based Health Services Management: a collaborating centre of the Joanna Briggs Institute, National Healthcare Group, Singapore
- Tzu Chi College of Technology JBI Evidence Synthesis Group for Promoting Health and Better Care, Tzu Chi College of Technology, Hualien, Taiwan
- Taiwan Joanna Briggs Institute Collaborating Centre, Taiwan: a collaborating centre of the Joanna Briggs institute, National Yang-Ming University, Taipei, Taiwan
- Joanna Briggs Institute Evidence Synthesis Group, Mahidol University, Bangkok, Thailand
- Thailand Centre for Evidence-Based Nursing and Midwifery: a collaborating centre of the Joanna Briggs Institute, Chiang Mai University, Chiang Mai, Thailand

Europe

- Thames Valley Centre for Evidence-Based Nursing and Midwifery: a collaborating centre of the Joanna Briggs Institute, Thames Valley University, London, England

- University of Nottingham Centre for Evidence-Based Nursing and Midwifery: a collaborating centre of the Joanna Briggs Institute, University of Nottingham, Nottingham, England
- Romanian Centre for Evidence-Based Public Health: a collaborating centre of the Joanna Briggs Institute, National School of Public Health and Health Services Management, Bucharest, Romania
- Scottish Centre for Evidence-Based Multi-Professional Practice: a collaborating centre of the Joanna Briggs Institute, Robert Gordon University, Aberdeen, Scotland
- Scottish Centre for Evidence-Based Care of Older People: a collaborating centre of the Joanna Briggs Institute, Glasgow Caledonian University, Glasgow, Scotland
- Spanish Centre for Evidence-Based Nursing: a collaborating centre of the Joanna Briggs Institute, Institute of Health Carlos III, Madrid, Spain
- Wales Centre for Evidence-Based Care: a collaborating centre of the Joanna Briggs Institute, Nursing Health and Social Care Research Centre, School of Nursing and Midwifery, Cardiff University, Cardiff, Wales

CHAPTER 2

Using the right type of evidence to answer clinical questions

Adrian Esterman, Jane Warland and Kate Deuter

2.1 Learning objectives

After reading this chapter, you should be able to:

1. understand the different types of research designs
2. discuss what constitutes quantitative, qualitative and mixed-method research and the evidence they produce
3. understand the use of hierarchies of evidence, and
4. describe the relationship between clinical question type and the source and type of study required to answer it.

2.2 Introduction

Broadly speaking, research designs can be divided into quantitative and qualitative. Quantitative research designs are based on measuring or counting things. They may be used to describe populations numerically; for example, to determine the average age of the population or the percentage who smoke. They are also designed to provide answers to questions, in other words to test hypotheses. Philosophically, quantitative research designs use a deductive approach; that is, they start with a statistical model and use the data collected to accept or reject the model. Quantitative research is designed to eliminate bias, or at least reduce it through the design itself or by statistical analysis. For this reason, quantitative researchers stand back from the research to ensure that they themselves do not introduce their own biases. Quantitative research is designed to be generalisable by use of a sufficiently large and representative sample.

Qualitative research is in many ways the opposite. It is based on natural enquiry, for example, observing or interviewing people. Rather than trying to answer a question, qualitative research is designed to explore the meaning of things. For example, a quantitative study might ask the question 'does this treatment work?', whereas a qualitative study might ask 'why does this treatment work and in what circumstances?' Qualitative research usually employs an inductive approach in that it moves from the data collected to a theory. Qualitative researchers often immerse themselves in the research, since elimination of bias is not a primary aim.

When designing a study, we usually start off with a research question followed by a series of aims, each addressing different aspects of the research question. It is the research question and study aims that determine whether a quantitative or qualitative approach should be used. For example, if the research question is 'how do people feel when their lifetime partner is diagnosed with a terminal illness?', then a qualitative approach is most suited to address this issue. Alternatively, if the research question is 'do hip protectors reduce fracture rates in elderly people?', then a quantitative approach is preferable. It is becoming increasingly common to see mixed approaches taken, where both qualitative and quantitative research are combined in a single study.

2.3 Quantitative research designs

2.3.1 Epidemiology

In many studies, the main aim is to determine whether exposure to a risk factor or health intervention is associated with a disease outcome. The scientific discipline that explores these relationships is called epidemiology. Epidemiology is the discipline underlying much of public health and clinical research, and is the foundation for much of the 'evidence' in evidence-based practice (EBP).

Every individual is unique; however, many individuals share common characteristics. For example, some drink or smoke, others may work in the same industry. Quite often the common characteristic is residing in the same city. It is the study of health in populations of people that differentiates epidemiology from clinical medicine, the latter being concerned with the study of health in individuals.

Last's *Dictionary of Epidemiology* describes epidemiology as 'the study of the distribution and determinants of health-related states or events in specified populations, and the application of this study to control of health problems' (Last 2000:62).

The distribution part of the statement refers to who contracts or suffers from the disease. For example, which age or gender groups are most affected? When did they get the disease? In which place or location did the disease occur? Determinants refer to what caused the disease. The study of disease causation is also known as aetiology.

Last (2000) uses the expression 'health-related states or events' since epidemiology now covers a wide range of health or health-related outcomes. In the earliest days of epidemiology, the main concern was study of infectious diseases. As these were gradually brought under control, attention then moved to acute diseases such as heart disease and cancer. More recently, we have focused on chronic diseases such as asthma and diabetes. We also now give priority to mental health problems, such as depression, and measures of quality of life. Finally, we are also interested in events such as accidents or birth defects. Clearly our understanding of disease has become much broader over time and this has shaped research.

Whenever we measure disease, we always do so with respect to the population at risk. For example, we might make the statement 'there were 1700 new cases of prostate cancer in Australian males in 2006'. We chose the male population since only males can get prostate cancer. The male population would be the estimated mid-year male resident population as at 30 June 2006.

In epidemiological studies, one of the primary goals is to measure the association between exposure to a risk factor (or health intervention) and disease—the stronger this association, the more likely the relationship to be causal. Two commonly used measures are the relative risk and the odds ratio. The relative risk (also known as the rate ratio) is calculated by dividing the percentage of people with the disease in the group exposed to the risk factor by the percentage of people with the disease in the group not exposed to the risk factor. Thus, a relative risk of 2 would be interpreted as those exposed to the risk factor would be twice as likely to get the disease as those not exposed to the risk factor. The odds ratio is a similar measure based on odds rather than on the percentage with the disease.

Finally, clinical epidemiology is the branch of epidemiology related to the use of epidemiological methods in patient populations. Importantly, this includes clinical trials of new drugs or health interventions. It is clinical epidemiology that underpins much of the high-level evidence for clinical interventions.

2.3.2 Sampling error

With quantitative research, we are nearly always working with samples of the population of interest rather than the whole population. We then make the major assumption that the conclusions drawn from our study are applicable to the whole population of interest, a process known as 'inference'. Sampling error is error due to the use of a sample rather than the whole population. Imagine that you had a ward of 30 patients and were trying to determine their average age. If you chose two patients at random and asked them their age, and then took the average, it would likely not be an accurate reflection of the true average age of the whole ward. However, if you took a sample of 10 patients at random, then the average age would likely be much closer to the true value. Thus, sampling error can be reduced by increasing the sample size.

2.3.3 Bias

Bias is defined as a consistent deviation from the truth. More formally, it is defined as 'deviation of results or inferences from the truth or processes leading to such deviation' (Last 2000). There are dozens of different types of potential bias, including bias relating to the collection, analysis, interpretation, publication or review of data (Last 2000). With respect to quantitative studies, the main biases of interest include:

- *Sampling bias*: bias due to the use of a non-random sample.
- *Ascertainment bias*: bias due to a failure to represent equally all classes of persons supposed to be represented (e.g. the use of electronic white pages to recruit subjects omits those who do not have a landline telephone).
- *Selection bias*: error due to systematic differences in characteristics between those who take part in a study and those who do not (e.g. volunteers might differ from non-volunteers).
- *Recall bias*: systematic differences in the accuracy of memory (e.g. people with mesothelioma—a cancer of the lining of the lung—are probably more likely to remember any exposure to asbestos).
- *Confounding bias*: this will be described in Section 2.3.5.

Unlike sampling error, bias cannot be reduced by increasing the sample size. One feature of quantitative studies are type I and II errors. A type I error occurs when the researcher, based on the study results, declares a treatment to be effective when it really is not. This is most often due to some type of bias. On the other hand, a type II error occurs when, based on the study results, a researcher declares a treatment to not be effective when it really is. This most often occurs when the researcher has used too small a sample size. In this case, the study is said to be underpowered.

2.3.4 Validity

The validity of a study (the word validity comes from the Latin *validus*, meaning strong) is the degree to which inferences or conclusions drawn from the study are warranted (Last 2000). We distinguish between internal and external validity. Internal validity is where any differences in outcome between study groups (apart from sampling error) can only be attributed to the hypothesised effect under investigation; in other words, the study is unbiased. External validity refers to how well it is possible to generalise the conclusions drawn from a study to other populations.

2.3.5 Confounding

Confounding is a special type of bias in which a measure of the effect of an exposure on risk is distorted because of the association of exposure with other factor(s) that influence the outcome under study (Last 2000). For example, in 1971, a case-control study by Cole found a link between coffee consumption and bladder cancer. In other words, the more coffee you drank, the more likely you were to get bladder cancer. However, it was later shown that heavy coffee drinkers were also more likely to smoke cigarettes, and it was the cigarette smoking causing the bladder cancer rather than the coffee drinking. Here we say that cigarette smoking confounds the relationship between coffee drinking and bladder cancer.

2.3.6 Randomised controlled trials

A randomised controlled trial (RCT) is the main type of experimental epidemiological study. In such a trial, subjects are randomly chosen from a population under investigation. One of the simplest possible study designs is the pre-post intervention study shown in Figure 2.1.

The key question here is whether any change in outcome at Time 2 has been caused by the intervention. Unfortunately, people tend to change naturally over time—something we call maturation bias—and therefore any changes observed at Time 2 might not have been caused by the intervention. Another potential cause of change over time unrelated to the intervention is regression to the mean. Regression to the mean is a statistical artifact where if a subject has a very high or low value of the outcome measure at Time 1, then they are likely to be closer to the mean value at Time 2.

To eliminate maturation bias and regression to the mean, we can introduce a control group who do not receive the intervention (see Fig 2.2).

Now if we compare the change in outcome from Time 1 to Time 2 between the intervention and control groups, we clearly have controlled for any possible maturation bias or regression to the mean.

Although the controlled pre-post intervention study is clearly a stronger design (i.e. less biased), it still has one major flaw. If the intervention and control groups have different characteristics at Time 1, then there is a strong possibility of confounding bias. For example, the intervention group might be older, and age could be a confounding factor. To reduce the possibility of confounding, we can randomise subjects into the two groups. Randomisation ensures that at Time 1 the two groups are well balanced with respect to population characteristics such as age, gender and severity of illness. This randomised controlled pre-post intervention study is more commonly known as an RCT. It appears near the top of tables of levels of evidence because the use of a control group and randomisation into intervention and control groups eliminates most types of bias.

Because the RCT is considered to be the 'gold standard' of study designs, a number of organisations have been formed to review and collate the evidence for different

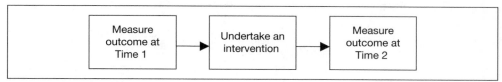

Figure 2.1 Pre-post intervention study

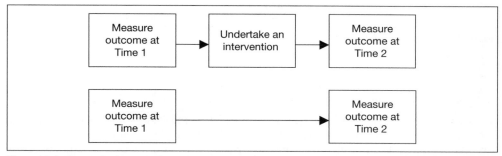

Figure 2.2 Controlled pre-post intervention study

interventions, focusing particularly on RCTs. This evidence is then stored in databases, including the:

- Cochrane Library (for general medical studies; see www.cochrane.org.au/library)
- PEDro database (for physiotherapy studies; see www.pedro.org.au), and
- Joanna Briggs database (for nursing studies; see www.joannabriggs.edu.au/about/home.php).

We have already seen how randomly allocating patients to study groups reduces potential confounding bias. Ideally, patients, researchers and those assessing the outcomes should not know to which group each patient has been assigned. This is known as blinding. Research has shown that non-blinded studies are more likely to show a treatment effect; that is, they are likely to suffer from bias. Medical journals have liaised and established a standardised format for reporting the results of RCTs—this is known as the Consolidated Standards of Reporting Trials (CONSORT) statement (see www.consort-statement.org). Researchers undertaking RCTs must first register their study protocol with a national registry of clinical trials (e.g. the Australian New Zealand Clinical Trials Registry; see www.anzctr.org.au/default.aspx) and then ensure that the paper presenting the results of the study exactly follows the CONSORT layout. This makes it easier for people undertaking systematic reviews to combine the results from different studies, a process known as meta-analysis. Registration of clinical trials also helps guard against publication bias; namely, that studies with positive results are more likely to be published than those with negative results.

2.3.7 Observational studies

There are many situations in which it is not ethical or even possible to undertake a randomised trial. For example, if you were interested in the relationship between marijuana use and schizophrenia, you could not ethically randomise subjects into those who must smoke marijuana and those who must not! In this type of situation, rather than deliberately expose people to a risk factor or intervention, we simply observe whether they have exposed themselves to it—hence the name 'observational' studies. The most commonly conducted observational studies are detailed on the next pages.

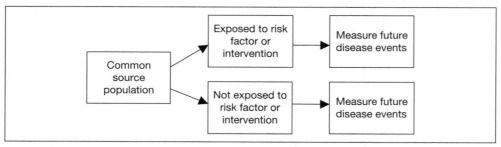

Figure 2.3 Cohort study

2.3.7.1 **Cohort studies**

Cohort studies investigate the association between people exposed to a risk factor or intervention and those not exposed, and the subsequent development of disease. All subjects belong to the one defined source population or cohort. Cohort studies begin with an exposed and a non-exposed group and follow them over time to see who develops different diseases. The study design may be prospective (from now into the future) or retrospective (from the past until now). Figure 2.3 shows this in diagrammatic form.

Since subjects are not randomised into groups, it is likely that the exposed and non-exposed groups are dissimilar at the start of the study and, hence, the study is open to confounding. Confounding factors therefore need to be identified and adjusted for during the statistical analysis. Cohort studies tend to be time consuming and expensive. They are not particularly useful for rare conditions, since you could follow many people for years and only end up with a handful of cases. Notably, cohort designs allow several types of disease or outcome measures to be assessed simultaneously.

2.3.7.2 **Case-control studies**

A case-control study design begins with a population of similar people. From this population, people with the disease (cases) and those without the disease (controls) are compared with respect to what risk factors each group was exposed to in the past. This either involves retrospectively examining records such as case notes and employment records, or asking participants to retrospectively recall details of their case through survey or interview. However, this can be problematic if the patient has died, and sometimes a proxy, such as the surviving spouse, is asked to complete the questionnaire. As previously mentioned, the main problem with a study of this type is with recall bias, where the participant cases are more likely to recall the exposure than the controls who do not have the disease and may not be aware of the risk factors and potential confounding variables. Figure 2.4 provides a diagram of the case-control study.

Both cases and controls should come from the same underlying target population. The ideal control group is one in which the control individuals are identical to the cases, apart from the fact that they do not have the disease. One way of ensuring this similarity is by matching cases and controls by potential confounding factors such as age, gender and socioeconomic status. Matching may occur by group or at the individual level. Case-control studies are cheaper and quicker to undertake than cohort studies. They also allow us to study several risk factors or exposures simultaneously. However, because of the problem of recall bias, they are placed lower in tables of levels of evidence than cohort studies.

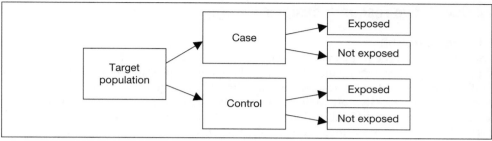

Figure 2.4 Case-control study

2.3.7.3 Cross-sectional studies

In a cross-sectional study, we interview a group of people to determine whether or not they have both a risk factor and disease at the same time. For example, we might be interested in where people work and whether or not they have respiratory problems. Since cross-sectional studies are not designed to provide information about time considerations (e.g. the risk factor or exposure could have occurred after the onset of health problems), they are considered to be a weaker design than cohort or case-control studies.

2.3.7.4 Ecological studies

Ecological studies are investigations using analyses of aggregated data. An example of an ecological study may be to investigate the correlation between data on diet and gastric cancer in different countries, and where the data are only available at the country level. Ecological studies suffer from the ecologic fallacy; that is, that associations found in aggregate data may not apply to individuals. In the above example, an association might be found between eating smoked food and gastric cancer; however, this association might not necessarily be true for any individual.

2.3.7.5 Case series

As its name implies, this type of study is where a series of cases are followed up to examine the natural history of a disease and to explore characteristics of cases for causal hypotheses. Case series are often undertaken by individual clinicians using their own patients, but can be undertaken at a population-wide level in the case of disease registries.

2.3.7.6 Hybrid designs

A number of other study designs that are variants of case-control studies are now being commonly used. These include:

- *Nested case-control studies*: these refer to a case-control study set within a cohort study. For example, when following a large cohort of women for incidence of breast cancer, Benichou et al (1997) drew a case-control subset from their larger cohort in order to examine the effects of mammographic features on breast cancer risk.
- *Case-cohort studies*: these also sit within a parent cohort study, but rather than taking matched controls for each case, a random subset of the initial cohort is used. The advantage of this design is that it allows both reuse of controls for different disease outcomes and estimation of the prevalence of exposure.
- *Case-crossover studies*: in this design, the case subjects act as their own control. Case-crossover designs are used where the risk factor or exposure is transient. For example, the relationship between long-haul flights and deep vein thrombosis was investigated with a case-crossover study (Kelman et al 2003).

2.4 Qualitative research designs

2.4.1 Introduction

For many nurses, the term 'evidence-based practice' suggests that the evidence required for informing clinical and policy decisions is based on empirical or quantitative research findings and, in particular, results from the 'pre-eminent gold standards' of systematic reviews and RCTs (Rycroft-Malone et al 2004). However, qualitative research can 'contribute substantially and in different ways to appropriateness of care' (Grypdonck 2006:1379). This section introduces the field of qualitative research and suggests ways in which nurses can identify and incorporate qualitative research evidence into their practice to maximise the chances that the care they deliver will be appropriate.

2.4.2 What is qualitative research?

A useful starting point in a discussion about qualitative research is to establish what it is not. A central feature of qualitative research is that it does not generate answers to research questions that are based on numbers. It has been widely argued that the qualitative researcher views the world through a very different lens—a view that is based upon the belief that there is no one singular universal truth; that the social world is multifaceted. In their discussion of issues regarding definition, Denzin and Lincoln (2005:3) describe qualitative research in the following way:

> ...qualitative research is a situated activity that locates an observer in the world. It consists of a set of interpretive, material practices that make the world visible. These practices transform the world. They turn the world into a series of representations, including field notes, interviews, conversations, photographs, recordings, and memos to the self. At this level, qualitative research involves an interpretive, naturalistic approach to the world. This means that qualitative researchers study things in their natural settings, attempting to make sense of, or interpret, phenomena in terms of the meanings people bring to them.

2.4.3 Methodology

It must be acknowledged that the field of qualitative research represents a diverse cluster of methodologies. An in-depth discussion of all of these is outside the scope of this text. In this section, we describe three common qualitative research methodologies that nurses use: ethnography, phenomenology and grounded theory.

2.4.3.1 Ethnography

Ethnography, the primary method of anthropology, is the earliest distinct tradition of qualitative inquiry (Patton 2002:81). Ethnographers study cultural behaviours, cultural knowledge and cultural artefacts in their search for cultural knowledge or understanding (Fitzgerald & Field 2005). Culture in an ethnographic study is not necessarily understood only as the study of a particular nation or ethnic group, so much as a group of people who have some kind of culture in common. For example, a recently published ethnographic study examined a group of critical care nurses and the role of technology in critical care nursing (Crocker & Timmons 2009). Focused clinical ethnographic studies provide important information about the ways in which the lives of patients and nurses intersect. Such understandings are important because they enable nurses to support patients through a deeper understanding of health and illness experiences.

2.4.3.2 Phenomenology

Qualitative researchers adopting a phenomenological approach seek to gain a deeper understanding of the nature or meaning of everyday 'lived' experiences of people (Van Manen 1990). The particular phenomenon may be one of many things—an emotion or a relationship, or it may be a program, an organisation or a culture (Patton 2002). Researchers who use this approach typically begin a research interview with a question such as 'what is your experience of...?' By gathering accounts of others' experiences, this information can be used to raise awareness of an impending intervention or circumstance (Fitzgerald & Field 2005). The strength of a phenomenological study is that it allows a person who has not had the experience to understand something about the essence of the experience through the participant's eyes. It is therefore useful to read phenomenological research reports as they may enable nurses to gain some empathy for their clients.

2.4.3.3 Grounded theory

While ethnography and phenomenology both focus on particular aspects of human experience, grounded theory focuses on the process of generating theory rather than a particular theoretical content (Patton 2002). In other words, there is no attempt in grounded theory studies to apply a conceptual framework before data are collected (Fitzgerald & Field 2005). Rather, data are analysed using a technique called 'constant comparative method'. This is where the researcher constantly compares emerging data for categories and constructs. Theory is thus grounded in the emergent data and is used to account for behavioural variation.

2.4.4 What do qualitative researchers do?

Qualitative researchers often begin their research with a general exploratory question and preliminary ideas. Following the collection of relevant data, they observe patterns in the data, organise these into a conceptual framework, and resume data collection to explore and challenge their developing conceptualisations (Russell et al 2005). Data are collected on multiple aspects of a study setting in order to assemble a broad and complete picture of the social dynamic of that setting (Litva & Jacoby 2007). Human-to-human methods include interviewing, participant and non-participant observation and focus groups. Artefactual 'text' methods include the use of documents such as letters, memoranda, reports and diaries (Litva & Jacoby 2007). Nursing 'texts' might include medical charts, journals and correspondence. Analysis of the data involves identifying recurring themes or patterns, and constructing a framework for communicating what is revealed (Patton 2002).

2.5 Triangulation and mixed-method studies

Triangulation was first described by Denzin (1978) as combining data sources to examine the phenomena of interest. Contrary to what the word may suggest, there do not have to be three sources of data in order for triangulation to occur. The aim of data triangulation is to provide data from two or more perspectives because this will inevitably increase understanding of the phenomena of interest. For example, in a study exploring the physiological and behavioural indicators of pain in neonates, data collection was triangulated to include data from nurse clinicians, pain researchers and the neonates themselves (Stevens et al 2009).

When multiple methods are used, the study is termed a mixed-methods study. Mixed-method studies commonly combine quantitative and qualitative data-collection approaches. A wide variety of methodological combinations can be employed to illuminate a research question (Patton 2002). For example, a study may include a single overarching methodology but use mixed methods for collecting the data (DiCenso et al 2005), or a researcher may combine two different methodological approaches, such as ethnography and interpretive phenomenology (Maggs-Rapport 2000). When combined with quantitative methods, qualitative approaches can be used to identify appropriate variables to be measured or questions to be asked. Insights from qualitative data can help to develop quantitative instruments that are more sensitive to respondents' meanings and interpretations (Coyle & Williams 2000).

2.6 Hierarchies of evidence

2.6.1 The strength of evidence

How do we judge how unbiased any given evidence is? With respect to evidence from scientific studies, certain types of study are designed to minimise bias. For example, an RCT uses a control group to guard against maturation bias as well as randomisation to remove the effect of confounding variables. Other study designs such as prospective cohort studies are less successful at minimising bias, but are still likely to be less biased than, say, expert opinion. Hence, textbooks on EBP invariably contain a hierarchy of levels of evidence, with systematic reviews of RCTs at the top and expert opinion at the bottom, the ordering being determined by the amount of perceived bias in the study design. Table 2.1 shows a table of levels of evidence provided by the National Health and Medical Research Council (NHMRC 2008).

2.6.2 Hierarchies of evidence and qualitative research

In comparison with quantitative research, many have argued that qualitative research lacks rigour and legitimacy, resulting in findings that have limited generalisability. As a consequence, qualitative research is either absent as a form of evidence or poorly ranked in methodological hierarchies of scientific evidence (Upshur 2001). Qualitative approaches are listed lower in these hierarchies because they are considered weak designs for addressing questions of effectiveness or causation. As a case in point, the Cochrane

Level of evidence	Study designs
I	Evidence obtained from a systematic review or meta-analysis of all relevant randomised controlled trials
II	Evidence obtained from at least one properly designed randomised controlled trial
III-1	Evidence obtained from well-designed pseudo-randomised controlled trials (alternate allocation or some other method)
III-2	Evidence obtained from comparative studies with concurrent controls and allocation not randomised (cohort studies), case-control studies, or interrupted time series without a parallel control group
III-3	Evidence obtained from comparative studies with historical control, two or more single-arm studies, or interrupted time series without a parallel control group
IV	Evidence obtained from case series (with either post-test or pre-test/post-test outcomes)

Table 2.1 Grading of research studies that measure the effect of an intervention, treatment or therapy
Source: NHMRC 2008

Collaboration (a highly regarded source that houses the highest level of research evidence) has struggled to find ways of incorporating evidence from qualitative research into systematic reviews. However, articles reporting qualitative systematic reviews are gradually beginning to make an appearance (Daly et al 2007). For example, Price (2009) conducted a meta-study of 10 qualitative studies in order to gain deep insight into the experience of choosing nursing as a career.

In qualitative research, concern about assessing quality is evident in both the proliferation of guidelines for performing and judging qualitative work, and the debates surrounding the nature of the knowledge produced by qualitative research approaches and how such research should be judged (Mays & Pope 2000). An important question for nurses is whether the quality of a research study can be legitimised and, if so, how. While the term 'rigour' often refers to discussions about objectivity, neutrality, reliability, replication and validity, a rigorous research approach essentially means that all the decisions made were well considered with alternatives and ramifications thought through (Steeves 2000).

Qualitative research is generally not designed to minimise or reduce bias, and it is for this reason that it is often not included in tables of levels of evidence. However, Daly et al (2007) have developed their own hierarchy of evidence for qualitative research, with individual case studies at the base and generalisable studies at the peak. Table 2.2 summarises the key features of each research approach.

Study type	Features	Limitations	Evidence for practice
Generalisable studies (level I)	Sampling focused by theory and the literature, extended as a result of analysis to capture diversity of experience. Analytic procedures comprehensive and clear. Located in the literature to assess relevance to other settings.	Main limitations are in reporting when the word length of articles does not allow a comprehensive account of complex procedures.	Clear indications for practice or policy may offer support for current practice, or critique with indicated directions for change.
Conceptual studies (level II)	Theoretical concepts guide sample selection, based on analysis of literature. May be limited to one group about which little is known or a number of important subgroups. Conceptual analysis recognises diversity in participants' views.	Theoretical concepts and minority or divergent views that emerge during analysis do not lead to further sampling. Categories for analysis may not be saturated.	Weaker designs identify the need for further research on other groups, or urge caution in practice. Well-developed studies can provide good evidence if residual uncertainties are clearly identified.
Descriptive studies (level III)	Sample selected to illustrate practical rather than theoretical issues. Record a range of illustrative quotes including themes from the accounts of 'many', 'most' or 'some' study participants.	Do not report full range of responses. Sample not diversified to analyse how or why differences occur.	Demonstrate that a phenomenon exists in a defined group. Identify practice issues for further consideration.
Single case studies (level IV)	Provide rich data on the views or experiences of one person. Can provide insights in unexplored contexts.	Do not analyse applicability to other contexts.	Alert practitioners to the existence of an unusual phenomenon.

Table 2.2 A hierarchy of evidence-for-practice in qualitative research: Summary features
Source: Daly et al 2007

The use of a hierarchy such as this can be viewed as both contentious and even pointless—contentious because qualitative researchers resent their research being ranked and compared in such a quantitative scale; pointless because there are circumstances where a single case study or a descriptive study is exactly what is needed to describe the phenomenon of interest and should therefore be the method of choice. Some of these points of contention have been resolved with the advent of triangulation and mixed-method studies.

There are a number of clear roles where qualitative research has been shown to be an essential part of providing evidence for treatment, including questionnaire design, interpreting results and answering questions about the impact, appropriateness and acceptability of interventions from the client's perspective. These roles and others are currently being explored by the Cochrane Qualitative Research Methods Group (see www.joannabriggs.edu.au/cqrmg). Qualitative design is flexible and has the capacity for adaptation to a wide range of research settings; however, it is this same flexibility that generates a range of study designs not easily captured in a single set of quality criteria (Daly et al 2007). This presents a challenge for nurses who wish to interpret results from studies conducted within the qualitative paradigm. While we acknowledge that the results of qualitative research can be used as an essential part of evidence-based practice, they should not be viewed as a substitute for quantitative research. Rather, quantitative research can most often be used as a basis for EBP, whereas results from qualitative studies inform the appropriateness of nursing practice. In this way, one complements the other.

2.7 Formulating the right question

Now that you understand the types of studies that nurses can conduct, we can move on to how nurses go about formulating research questions. This is important because you can't begin to look for an answer unless you have asked the right question.

Using the hierarchies of evidence introduced earlier in this chapter, we can examine some research questions and the ways we might find answers. The research questions and corresponding methods described in Table 2.3 are offered as a broad overview of some of the types of questions nurses may ask and the type of study required to answer each type of question.

What study type would you use to answer the following questions:

1. Does wearing a surgical face mask reduce postoperative infection?
2. What is it like to care for a partner with Alzheimer's disease?

The first question is aimed at discovering how effective surgical face masks are in reducing infection rates. Using the table below we can see that this question could be

Type of question	Type of method
How prevalent is this condition?	Survey
What is the effect of an intervention?	Randomised controlled trial
What is the effect of an exposure?	Cohort
What is the cause of a disease?	Case-control
Are the exposure and condition related?	Cross-sectional
How do people feel about their condition or treatment?	Qualitative

Table 2.3 Finding the best evidence by using the correct study type

answered by using a cohort study; for example, comparing postoperative infection rates between two theatres—one where all staff wore masks and one where they did not. The table indicates that the second question can best be answered by a qualitative study where, for example, you would interview partners of people with Alzheimer's disease.

These examples demonstrate that just as the first question cannot adequately be answered by interviewing staff about their *feelings* concerning mask wearing in theatre, neither can the second question be answered by comparing *numbers* of partners who care for people with Alzheimer's disease with partners of people with another related disorder.

Now let's briefly discuss how you might develop your own focused research question. The PICO (Patient Intervention Comparison Outcome) strategy identified by Sackett et al (1997) and Strauss et al (2005) can assist you in framing your question in terms of the relationship between its clearly defined parts. For example, questions addressing quantitative information (i.e. information about the effectiveness of an intervention or treatment) would typically consist of the following parts: the *population* (patient population), an *intervention* (such as a treatment, diagnostic test or treatment procedure), a *comparison intervention* (if any) and the *outcome* of the intervention. Questions requiring qualitative information would typically consist of two parts: the *population* (patient population) and the *situation* (condition, experiences or circumstances). Chapter 5 delivers a more comprehensive discussion around developing research questions (using the PICO strategy), as well as searching for and appraising high-quality evidence.

2.8 Conclusion

This chapter has introduced epidemiology as the underpinning discipline of quantitative design and the foundation upon which 'evidence' in EBP is grounded. This was followed by a synopsis of quantitative and qualitative research designs. As shown, the unique characteristics of both quantitative and qualitative research approaches can be combined to enable nurses to locate the highest quality research evidence available. This is clearly evident in the increasing prevalence of mixed-method and triangulated studies. Regardless of the type of research employed, high-level evidence emerges from systematic studies that employ rigorous research design, data collection, interpretation and communication. Nurses need to look for these signposts when searching for evidence to address clinical questions.

2.9 DISCUSSION QUESTIONS

1. Describe three patient-centred issues you have encountered recently and turn them into questions. What types of questions are they?
2. For each of the questions, describe the types of study you would search for to find an answer to your question.
3. The NHMRC (2008) has produced 'Levels of evidence' tables. They are only useful for evaluating particular study types. What types of studies are these?
4. Discuss the challenges associated with the inclusion of qualitative research in hierarchies of evidence.

2.10 **References**

Australian New Zealand Clinical Trials Registry. Available: www.anzctr.org.au/default.aspx 27 Apr 2009.

Benichou J, Byrne C, Gail M 1997 An approach to estimating exposure-specific rates of breast cancer from a two-stage case-control study within a cohort. *Statistics in Medicine* 16(1–3):133–51.

Cochrane Library. Available: www.cochrane.org.au/library 25 Apr 2009.

Cochrane Qualitative Research Methods Group. Available: www.joannabriggs.edu.au/cqrmg 27 Apr 2009.

Cole P 1971 Coffee-drinking and cancer of the lower urinary tract. *Lancet* 1(7713):1335–7.

CONSORT statement. Available: www.consort-statement.org 27 Apr 2009.

Coyle J, Williams B 2000 An exploration of the epistemological intricacies of using qualitative data to develop a quantitative measure for user views of health care. *Journal of Advanced Nursing* 31(5):1235–43.

Crocker C, Timmons S 2009 The role of technology in critical care nursing. *Journal of Advanced Nursing* 65(1):52–61.

Daly J, Willis K, Small R et al 2007 A hierarchy of evidence for assessing qualitative health research. *Journal of Clinical Epidemiology* 60(1):43–9.

Denzin N K 1978 *The research act: a theoretical introduction to sociological methods, 2nd edn.* McGraw-Hill, New York.

Denzin N K, Lincoln Y S 2005 *The Sage handbook of qualitative research, 3rd edn.* Sage Publications, Thousand Oaks, CA.

DiCenso A, Hutchison B, Grimshaw J et al 2005 Health services interventions. In: DiCenso A, Guyatt G, Ciliska D (eds) *Evidence-based nursing: a guide to clinical practice.* Elsevier Mosby, St Louis, MO.

Fitzgerald M, Field J 2005 Qualitative research designs. In: Courtney M (ed) *Evidence for nursing practice.* Elsevier, Sydney.

Grypdonck M 2006 Qualitative health research in the era of evidence-based practice. *Qualitative Health Research* 16(10):1371–85.

Joanna Briggs database Available: www.joannabriggs.edu.au/about/home.php 19 May 2009.

Kelman C W, Kortt M A, Becker N G et al 2003 Deep vein thrombosis and air travel: record linkage study. *British Medical Journal* 327(7423):1072.

Last J M 2000 *A dictionary of epidemiology, 4th edn.* Oxford University Press, New York.

Litva A, Jacoby A 2007 Qualitative research: critical appraisal. In: Craig J V, Smyth R L (eds) *The evidence-based practice manual for nurses.* Churchill Livingstone, Edinburgh.

Maggs-Rapport F 2000 Combining methodological approaches in research: ethnography and interpretive phenomenology. *Journal of Advanced Nursing* 31(1):219–25.

Mays N, Pope C 2000 Qualitative research in health care: assessing quality in qualitative research. *British Medical Journal* 320(7226):50–2.

National Health and Medical Research Council (NHMRC) 2008 *NHMRC additional levels of evidence and grades for recommendations for developers of guidelines. Stage 2 Consultation 2008–2010.* NHMRC, Commonwealth of Australia, Canberra.

Patton 2002 *Qualitative research and evaluation methods.* Sage Publications, Thousand Oaks, CA.

PEDro database. Available: www.pedro.org.au 27 Apr 2009.

Price S 2009 Becoming a nurse: a meta-study of early professional socialization and career choice in nursing. *Journal of Advanced Nursing* 65(1):11–9.

Russell C, Gregory D, Ploeg J et al 2005 Qualitative research. In: DiCenso A, Guyatt G, Ciliska D (eds) *Evidence-based nursing: a guide to clinical practice.* Elsevier Mosby, St Louis, MO.

Rycroft-Malone J, Seers K, Tichen A et al 2004 What counts as evidence in evidence-based practice? *Journal of Advanced Nursing* 47(1):81–90.

Sackett D L, Richardson W S, Rosenberg W et al 1997 *Evidence-based medicine: how to practice and teach EBM.* Churchill Livingstone, New York, NY.

Steeves R 2000 Writing the results. In: Cohen M, Kahn D, Steeves R (eds) *Hermeneutic phenomenological research: a practical guide for nurse researchers.* Sage Publications, Thousand Oaks, CA.

Stevens B, McGrath P, Dupuis A et al 2009 Indicators of pain in neonates at risk for neurological impairment. *Journal of Advanced Nursing* 65(2):285–96.

Strauss S E, Richardson W S, Glazsiou P et al 2005 *Evidence-based medicine: how to practice and teach EBM, 3rd edn*. Elsevier Churchill Livingstone, Edinburgh.

Upshur R E G 2001 The status of qualitative research as evidence. In: Morse J M, Swanson J M, Kuzel AJ (eds) *The nature of qualitative evidence*. Sage Publications, Thousand Oaks, CA.

Van Manen M 1990 *Researching lived experience: human science for an action sensitive pedagogy*. Althouse Press, London.

PART TWO

Developing an evidence-based culture

CHAPTER 3

Developing a culture of inquiry to sustain evidence-based practice

Sonya Osborne and Glenn Gardner

3.1 Learning objectives

After reading this chapter, you should be able to:

1. describe important features of a culture of inquiry
2. conduct a self-assessment of your own organisation in relation to these features
3. discuss barriers that impede development of an evidence-based practice (EBP) culture and identify the presence of any of these barriers in your own organisation, and
4. apply a range of strategies or interventions, targeted at identified barriers, for developing a culture of inquiry and sustaining EBP, particularly those that may work in your organisation.

3.2 Introduction

> Culture does not change because we desire to change it. Culture changes when the organisation is transformed; the culture reflects the realities of people working together every day (Hesselbein 2002:2).

Evidence-based practice (EBP) is having a significant effect on the health service environment. It constructs a language that bridges the healthcare disciplines and the clinical and managerial components of health services. Most experienced clinicians in nursing, medicine and allied health now recognise that the contemporary healthcare environment calls for our practice to be justified by sound, credible evidence. There is pressure on all clinicians to accommodate innovation, while at the same time ensuring their practice is effective, safe and efficient (Forbes & Griffiths 2002). Consequently, EBP in healthcare is having a profound effect on nursing and the way we think about nursing.

There are many available models for research utilisation that are dependent on organisational strategies for change. This chapter describes the relationship between organisation and culture, and explores the notion of cultural change; that is, developing a culture of inquiry that can sustain EBP. We begin this chapter with a clear conception of what we mean by EBP and what we mean by 'culture'.

3.3 Evidence-based practice in healthcare

EBP has been thoroughly defined in Chapter 1. In summary, EBP is making clinical decisions using the best available evidence, in conjunction with clinical expertise, and judgment and knowledge of the patient. Essentially, EBP is about reducing uncertainty in clinical care, leading to efficient and effective service delivery. It is about asking questions of our practice, systematically searching for answers to these questions, applying the best possible evidence from this search at the clinical interface and then evaluating the effect of this evidence-informed care.

However, evidence-based decision making is not as easy as following a five- or six-step recipe. First, clinicians are not born with the skills to be evidence-based practitioners. Second, the 'evidence' is, quite often, inaccessible, unreadable, invalid, not available, not applicable or lacking in quality (Bryar et al 2003, Funk et al 1991, Kajermo et al 1998, Miller & Messenger 1978, Parahoo & McCaughan 2001, Retsas 2000). Although healthcare organisations acknowledge the promotion and support of EBP, few provide the infrastructure, resources, support and incentives necessary to develop and sustain a culture of inquiry (Osborne, unpublished work, 2009).

Tranmer et al (1998) suggest that i) there is lack of organisational support to develop EBP and research the utilisation knowledge and skills of nurse clinicians; and ii) in the absence of evidence, there is lack of organisational support to generate nurse-initiated evidence for practice through the conduct of research. Organisations that can enable the culture by building infrastructure and developing EBP competency in staff will create a professional practice environment that fosters personal and professional staff development as well as developments and improvements in the quality of care delivered to patients (Newhouse et al 2005, Newhouse 2007).

3.4 Culture and organisation in healthcare

In this chapter, we will take the anthropological view instead of the positivist view in defining what we mean by culture—that is, a discussion based on the premise that an organisation does not *have* a culture, it *is* a culture. A common expression defining culture in the healthcare environment is 'culture is the way we do things around here'. Others have defined culture more formally as:

> …a pattern of shared basic assumptions that the group learned as it solved
> its problems of external adaptation and internal investigation, that has
> worked well enough to be considered valid and, therefore, to be taught to new
> members as the correct way to perceive, think, and feel in relation to those
> problems (Schein 1992:12).

In any organisation, however, the organisational culture also contains a number of subcultures that ascribe to a pattern of basic assumptions based on a shared perspective. In healthcare, those shared perspectives can be based on discipline (e.g. nurses or medical doctors), gender, age, geographical location (e.g. ward or unit, acute facility or community outreach clinic), experience (e.g. novice nurses or expert nurses) or specialty field (e.g. acute care or critical care; orthopaedics or oncology). Supporting an organisational culture of inquiry happens in a cultural environment made up of individual clinicians and subgroups of individual clinicians, each with their own values, beliefs, assumptions and behaviours. Therefore, before we can expect an organisational cultural change, we must first effect an attitude change in the individual clinician. By making organisation synonymous with culture, cultural change involves altering or transforming the basic assumptions of the organisation. If the basic assumptions of the subcultures make up the organisational culture, then cultural change will have to begin with the subcultures and, more basically, with the individuals that make up the subcultures. Given that definitions determine actions, thoughts and perceptions (Bate 1994:9), we must conceptualise an evidence-based culture or, more aptly, *a culture of inquiry*, before we can discuss and recognise a 'cultural change'.

3.5 What is a culture of inquiry?

In order to transform organisational culture to one that values EBP, it is necessary to have a clear idea of what a culture of inquiry looks like. A culture of inquiry is a culture that supports clinicians in making healthcare decisions that are based upon finding and using the best available evidence and combining that with their clinical expertise and their knowledge of the patient to guide decision making in healthcare. An organisation that promotes a culture of inquiry must:

- develop clinicians who are capable of using the EBP process in their clinical practice
- provide resources for clinicians to be practitioners whose practice is underpinned by best available evidence, and
- give clinicians the autonomy, authority and control to participate collaboratively in healthcare decisions and effect change in their clinical practice based on best available evidence.

Learning has been described as being on a continuum, which, if reinforced over time, will lead to permanent changes in behaviour (Webb et al 1996). Thus, a culture of inquiry is a learning culture that encourages interrogation of practice by providing the necessary resources to formulate questions, search for answers and evaluate the answers in practice. Such a culture recognises the value of research and the integration of research findings into practice by providing the necessary infrastructure, resources, support and incentives to enable nurse clinicians to fully engage in the EBP agenda.

Healthcare occurs in a multidisciplinary and multidimensional environment. Therefore, a culture of inquiry tolerates diversity and promotes true collaboration in the decision-making process on issues regarding patient care. Such a culture also has particular attributes associated with a participative management, such as a flat versus hierarchical management framework and decentralised administration (Havens & Vasey 2003). Organisational strategies that enhance nurse involvement in decision making provide nurses with a voice in both patient care decisions and in nursing work decisions. Such involvement in decision making has implications for positive patient outcomes (Havens & Vasey 2003), such as lower patient morbidity and mortality (Aiken et al 1994, Baggs et al 1999), shorter mean length of stay (Aiken et al 1999), and fewer patient complaints (Havens 2001).

In addition to valuing collaboration and involvement in decision making, a culture of inquiry values and supports autonomy and authority in decision making in areas of expertise. Autonomy has been defined as 'an individual's ability to independently carry out the responsibilities of the position without close supervision' (Blanchfield & Biordi 1996:43). Authority has been defined as 'sanctioned or legitimate power to make decisions' (Blanchfield & Biordi 1996:43). Thus, a culture of inquiry recognises the legitimate authority of nurse clinicians, values professional nurse autonomy and encourages nurse involvement in healthcare decision making, thus providing support for change and innovation in practice.

There are benefits to having a culture of inquiry for both patients and nurses. It was demonstrated more than two decades ago that patients who are the recipients of nursing care that is based on research have better outcomes. Heater et al (1988) conducted a meta-analysis of nurse-conducted experimental research and found that patients who are the recipients of research-based nursing interventions can expect 28% better outcomes than patients who receive standard nursing care. This early study supports the assumption that engagement in the EBP and research agenda improves patient outcomes.

Benefits to nurses working in an organisation that values EBP and nurses' contribution to healthcare have also been demonstrated in the literature. Several authors reported strong associations between autonomous decision making in clinical practice, job satisfaction and perceived productivity in organisations where the nurse leader values education and professional development of all nurses (Kramer & Schmalenberg 2003a, 2003b; Scott et al 1999). EBP is a great equaliser because the role of authority and opinion is no longer a sufficient basis for decisions about healthcare (Osborne & Gardner 2004). Rather, rules of evidence take precedence in clinical decision making (Osborne & Gardner 2004).

Later in this chapter, we will describe two different systems designed to nurture a learning culture that values research, translation of research into practice, diversity, collaboration and autonomous decision making in order to develop and sustain a culture of inquiry; namely, Magnet Hospitals and Practice Development Units.

3.6 Development towards a culture of inquiry

Gaining and maintaining commitment to organisational change is critical to enhancing the chances of a successful change towards a culture of inquiry. Culture has been defined as a pattern of basic assumptions and values that an organisation shares. Thus, transforming into a culture of inquiry requires a change in the pattern of these basic assumptions and values. As an organisation is transformed into a culture of inquiry, clinical practice once guided by 'that's the way we do it around here' or 'that's the way we were told to do it' is replaced with clinical practice guided by the more questioning imperative of 'what's the evidence for that?'.

Organisational leaders must develop strategies to achieve a receptive context for the kind of culture and climate that supports and enables EBP, innovation and change (Greenhalgh et al 2004, Thiel & Ghosh 2008). Changing to a culture of inquiry can be problematic. Without simultaneous change at both the macro (organisation) level and micro (nurse clinician) level, cultural change will not be sustainable. Change in the culture of an organisation requires commitment to change by the individual members of the organisation's subcultures. However, to gain and maintain this commitment to change, the organisation must fully support its individual members throughout the change. Organisational support for a culture of inquiry is required to remove identified barriers to research utilisation, to build capacity to engage in the EBP agenda, and to encourage and support innovation in practice by recognising and supporting authority and autonomy for clinicians to effect practice change.

3.6.1 Removal of well-identified barriers

Research is still perceived by most nurse clinicians as external to practice, and implementing research findings into practice is often difficult. Barriers to research utilisation by nurses have been discussed in the international nursing literature for more than three decades (Bryar et al 2003, Funk et al 1991, Kajermo et al 1998, Miller & Messenger 1978,

Parahoo & McCaughan 2001, Retsas 2000). In 1978, the most frequent problems encountered when trying to put research findings in place included:
1. inability to obtain research findings in one's own area of interest
2. the time and costs involved in implementing research
3. resistance to change in the work setting
4. lack of relevance of the findings
5. lack of understanding or agreement with conclusions, and
6. lack of rewards for implementation (Miller & Messenger 1978).

Although the quantity and quality of nursing research has improved since then, the use of research findings in practice remains low. In 1991, Funk et al found the two greatest barriers reported by nurses were 'nurses not feeling they had enough authority to change patient care procedures' and 'insufficient time on the job to implement new ideas'. Both are barriers of the organisational setting (Funk et al 1991). Moreover, most of the other barriers in the 'top 10 list' were those related to the organisational setting, including lack of cooperation and support from physicians, other staff and administration, inadequate facilities for implementation, and insufficient time to read research (Funk et al 1991). Barriers reported in the past vary little from barriers reported today. In general, aspects of the organisational setting and aspects of the research itself continue to represent the greatest problem areas. Lack of time to read and apply findings, lack of organisational support, lack of peer support, and lack of authority to change practice continue to rank highest in the list (Brown et al 2009, Bryar et al 2003, Fink et al 2005, Kajermo et al 1998, Parahoo & McCaughan 2001, Retsas 2000). A recent integrative review of 45 studies using the BARRIERS Scale found no evidence to support the theory that the identification of barriers to nurses' use of research influenced nursing practice, and concluded that research is needed to investigate whether there is a relationship between perceptions of barriers and nurses' use of research and EBP (Carlson & Plonczynski 2008). To achieve successful cultural change towards a culture of inquiry, organisations must not only recognise these barriers but also put strategies in place to reduce or eliminate them.

3.6.2 Capacity building in evidence-based practice and research utilisation

Difficulty in not only understanding but also accepting research findings is widespread (Bryar et al 2003, Funk et al 1991, Kajermo et al 1998, Miller & Messenger 1978, Parahoo & McCaughan 2001, Retsas 2000), and presents a serious challenge for the promotion of EBP in nursing. This is an issue not easily solved and in part is related to the nursing culture. Nursing is an old profession. Our beginnings are steeped in rituals, traditions and folklore. Despite the fact that nursing has changed in recent years and the *context* of nursing practice has changed dramatically, for too many nurses these rituals, traditions and folklores persist (Holland 1993, O'Callaghan 2001, Strange 2002, Winslow 1998). This creates an environment that resists change, does not question and does not look to science to inform practice. In this environment, research skills will not be valued. In conjunction with this historical cultural background is the varying quality of research education in undergraduate nursing programs and varying support from organisations for postgraduate research training for nurses.

The skills necessary to conduct EBP are easily identified and relate to competencies such as searching and retrieval of research literature, critical appraisal of research reports, and a level of skill in the design and conduct of epidemiological research. The skills and attitudes necessary to sustain a culture of inquiry are less easy to acquire and have been identified as having a professional pride and vision to build the evidence base for practice, being motivated and having the willingness, energy, enthusiasm, tenacity and ability to initiate change, being aware of own strengths and limitations, and having commitment to continuous learning (Bland & Ruffin 1992, McCormack & Garbett 2003, Scott et al 1999). Clinical academic positions that are joint appointments between a tertiary institution and a healthcare facility can play a major role in achieving change in this area by role modelling, promoting collaboration, supporting change agents and empirically demonstrating the value of EBP.

It may seem simple enough to provide resources for the training programs and equipment needed to engage in EBP, but organisations have to do more. They have to provide an infrastructure that will not only sustain continual learning in EBP, but also support nurses in making changes based on the evidence. In most organisations, clinical practice consumes all of nursing time with little time and space for development of that practice through questioning practice, reading research, and initiating and implementing innovations in practice. In short, in the contemporary healthcare environment, there is insufficient time for nurses to engage in EBP.

The literature is clear that this is an organisational problem. The organisation needs to make time for nurses to develop their practice. However, organisational responsibility is only the first step. Time is a commodity in the clinical environment that is quickly consumed with patient care activities. For example, if an overlap time exists between shifts, this may well provide opportunity for nurses to plan new initiatives. However, what is likely to happen is that clinical care will encroach on this time. The work of patient care is unlimited and will expand to fill the time available. So, organisational responsibility is not the final answer. The challenge is for nurses to create their own time for interrogating, developing and changing practice.

After protected time for engaging in the EBP agenda is negotiated with nursing managers and made available through an organisational commitment to build time into existing work rosters, creation and protection of that time needs to come from the clinical staff. Teams must be facilitated to identify creative ways to ensure that negotiated time for developing practice is available. This requires a commitment from the whole team and a determination to own the problem and the solution. Nurse clinicians must collaborate with each other and take responsibility and control of their work environment to break down this time barrier.

Enabling EBP within organisations is important for promoting positive outcomes for nurses and patients. Fostering EBP is a long-term developmental process within organisations, not a static or immediate outcome (Newhouse et al 2005). Once the question of '*Why* aren't nurses using research?' is attended to and barriers are removed, organisations need to ask the questions, 'how?' and 'what?'. Implementation requires multiple strategies to cultivate a culture of inquiry where nurses generate and answer important questions to guide practice (Newhouse et al 2005). Organisations need to ask '*how* we can shift the culture forward beyond exploration and towards integration of evidence with decision making?' and '*what* do nurses need to effect change in practice?'

3.6.3 Support for autonomy and authority to change practice

Autonomy has been defined as 'an individual's ability to independently carry out the responsibilities of the position without close supervision' and 'is closely linked to authority' (Blanchfield & Biordi 1996:43). In a concept analysis of the plethora of literature on autonomy, Ballou (1998) found several emerging themes in the literature. Autonomy encompasses 'a self-governance system of principles, competence or capacity, decision-making, critical reflection, freedom, and self-control' (Ballou 1998:103). As previously mentioned, the literature demonstrates a strong association between autonomous decision making in clinical practice, job satisfaction and perceived productivity in organisations where the nurse leader values education and professional development of all nurses (Scott et al 1999), which are key requisites in capacity building in EBP.

There is typically a lack of decision-making power by nurses related to patient management issues within the medically dominated health system hierarchy. Nursing clinical practice and medical practice are perceived as linked. However, nursing practice is more likely to be seen as dependent upon medical decision making. This perception, at times, has the effect of subsuming nurse decision making and autonomy over nursing practice to a task-oriented role under the direction of medicine. Healthcare is multidisciplinary and decisions made about patient care should reflect a true collaborative relationship between disciplines by relinquishing control over aspects of patient care management to those disciplines that have legitimate responsibility for those aspects of care. Relationships focused on optimising patient outcomes should replace relationships based on power.

Literature abounds with alternative strategies, models, plans and algorithms for research utilisation, EBP, implementing practice change and getting clinicians to buy into the change (Kitson et al 1998, Newhouse et al 2005, Rosswurm & Larrabee 1999, Rycroft-Malone 2004, Stetler 2001, Stevens 2004, Titler et al 2001). Despite their abundance, however, there is limited evidence of effectiveness of these frameworks and models for change (Foxcroft et al 2009, Greenhalgh et al 2004). Models of change that encourage clinicians to become evidence-based practitioners and strategies for assisting such change usually hinge on the organisation committing more resources, more time and more development. This infrastructure enables the first three steps in the EBP process (i.e. formulate a question, find the evidence, appraise the evidence) to occur. It may not address the further steps of applying the evidence and evaluating the practice change. This may be effective for nurse-to-nurse buy-in, but what about cross-disciplinary buy-in? Even practices that nurses have control over are influenced by other disciplines.

One example of this is wound care. Wound care has been a responsibility of nursing since the time of Florence Nightingale. Nurses have managed wounds from pressure ulcers and vascular ulcers to postoperative wounds, post-radiation therapy wounds and ostomy wounds, but why don't nurses have autonomous control over choice of wound management interventions? Even where there is strong evidence favouring a particular wound dressing intervention, the nurse clinician often, in many settings, perceives that they do not have the autonomy or authority to make the decision to evaluate a practice change. Nurses need to seize back the requisite autonomy and authority to make practice change decisions based on evidence, without hindrance from medical determination. Here is the place where a cultural or organisational change is needed. There is no magic bullet to changing an organisation to a culture of inquiry, but if the organisation is going to espouse to being an EBP organisation, all clinicians must be able to change their practice based on the integration of best available evidence, clinician judgment and patient values. Only then can the organisation truly be a culture of inquiry.

The EBP movement has both great potential and challenges for the development of the discipline of nursing. The potential of EBP is in two main areas:
1. It provides a scientific framework for building the practice knowledge base for nursing.
2. If harnessed, EBP can support clinical autonomy and advanced practice roles for nursing.

Clinical autonomy or decision-making influence over one's own practice comes with confidence in the knowledge base of that practice. Nursing has undergone a dramatic change in the past 2–3 decades. In many countries, the education of nurses at some, if not all, levels is conducted in the tertiary environment. As a consequence, nursing has developed and continues to develop a knowledge base through research and scholarly inquiry. Additionally, there is a vast amount of skill, knowledge and expertise in nursing practice. Nursing is lifesaving, it is therapeutic, it is caring, it is scientific and it is technological. And nursing is central to the operation of healthcare. This has become more evident in the recent and continuing global nursing shortage, which has resulted in a crisis in many healthcare systems. Nursing has authority through its knowledge base, its expertise and its role in healthcare. The challenge for nurses in gaining autonomy to change practice is to continue to identify the domains of nursing practice and to systematically gather evidence to support best practice in these domains.

3.7 Culture of inquiry 'in action'

Attempts are being made to develop cultures of inquiry in healthcare using a variety of processes. Two examples, Magnet Hospitals, conceived and established in the USA, and Practice Development Units, established in the UK (although adopted and adapted in Australia), are described here to highlight similarities in the strategic aims, structure, processes and outcomes of each in establishing and maintaining a culture of inquiry in healthcare.

3.7.1 Magnet Hospitals

In 1982, the American Academy of Nursing (AAN) conducted its first 'Magnet' study to explore factors that affected recruitment and retention of professional nurses. The study found core organisational characteristics existed among 41 hospitals distinguished by high nurse satisfaction, low job turnover and low nurse vacancy rates (McClure et al 1983). The study found that an environment that supports nursing excellence was a key factor not only in attracting and retaining highly qualified nurses, but also in promoting positive patient care outcomes. Key characteristics of the original Magnet Hospitals included the following:

- a nurse executive was a formal member of the highest decision-making body in the organisation
- the nursing service was organised in a flat organisational structure
- decision making was decentralised to the unit level
- nurses on each unit were given responsibility for organising care and staffing appropriate to patient needs
- administrative structures supported nurses' decisions about care, and
- good communication existed between nurses and physicians (McClure et al 1983).

Today, the Magnet Hospital concept has been renewed and formalised in the Magnet Nursing Services Recognition Program™, which is administered by the American Nurses Credentialing Center (ANCC) and based on the American Nurses Association's nursing quality indicators and standards of nursing practice.

The overall goal of the program is to recognise excellence in the provision of quality nursing care and acknowledge organisations that 'uphold the tradition within nursing of professional nursing practice' (ANCC 2003). The program also provides a medium for disseminating successful practices and strategies among nursing services (ANCC 2003). There has been a significant amount of research on the Magnet Hospital concept as a model of professional nursing practice since its inception, demonstrating that Magnet Hospitals had better outcomes than non-Magnet Hospitals (McClure et al 1983, Scott et al 1999).

Subsequent research has highlighted other important characteristics that have an effect on recruitment and retention related to the hospital nurse leaders, such as: visibility and staff support; characteristics related to clinical nursing practice, such as autonomy and control within clinical practice, status within the organisation and collaboration across levels and disciplines; and characteristics related to the organisational culture, such as participative management and support of professional development (Kramer & Schmalenberg 2003a, 2003b; Scott et al 1999). Research suggests that Magnet Hospitals accredited under the ANCC program had even better outcomes than the original Magnet Hospitals (Scott et al 1999), and that there is an association between the characteristics of professional nursing as demonstrated in Magnet Hospitals and the impact on patient outcomes, such as morbidity, mortality and satisfaction with nursing care (Aiken et al 1994, Aiken et al 1997, Havens & Aiken 1999, Scott et al 1999, Turkel et al 2005).

In the original Magnet Hospitals study, outcomes were the variables evaluated as being able to differentiate Magnet Hospitals from non-Magnet Hospitals. These outcomes (i.e. structures, characteristics and attributes) were then used to generate structural characteristics of facilities perceived to be associated with the outcomes. Between 1989 and 1993, these characteristics of 'magnetism' were the focus of Magnet Hospital research; after 1993, Magnet Hospital research turned its attention towards evaluating foundational structural elements based on nurse administrators' scope of practice and 14 'forces of magnetism'(Kramer & Schmalenberg 2005:279) identified from the early studies. The 'forces of magnetism'—which continue to attract nursing staff in contemporary healthcare—relate to quality improvement, interdisciplinary relationships, professional models of care, consultation, resources, autonomy, the community and the hospital, nurses as teachers, the image of nursing, professional development, personnel policies and programs, the quality of nursing leadership, management style, and organisational structure (Kramer & Schmalenberg 2005).

The ANCC Magnet Nursing Services Recognition Program™ 'offers an evidence-based model for nurse leaders interested in transforming the practice climate' (Stolzenberger 2003:522). While the focus of Magnet Hospitals and the Magnet Hospital literature is on recruitment and retention of nurses, organisational characteristics aimed at improving recruitment and retention are key characteristics of organisations that support a culture of inquiry.

3.7.2 Practice Development Units

Another approach, which has grown in momentum over the past two decades and is aimed at supporting a culture of inquiry, is Practice Development. A Practice Development Unit has the potential to transcend the barriers to research utilisation in practice by strategically and systematically enhancing clinical effectiveness in patient health outcomes through best practice innovations, while stimulating a change in the culture and context of care (Manley & McCormack 2003).

Practice Development has its theoretical underpinning in critical social science. Critical social science is an attempt to understand in a rationally responsible manner the oppressive features of a society, so that this understanding stimulates its audience to transform their society and thereby liberate themselves (Fay 1987). In other words, Practice Development as a methodology aims to guide nurses away from the perception that they cannot make decisions and influence healthcare because of medical domination. The process takes them on a journey—from discovering the factors in their 'socioprofessional' environment that both inhibit and enable them to demonstrate their contribution to health outcomes, to feeling empowered to participate in healthcare decisions (Osborne 2009). This is achieved by enabling nurses with the skills to interrogate and change from a practice based on traditions, rituals and myths to a practice based on evidence. Practice Development has been defined in contemporary literature as:

> ... a continuous process of increased effectiveness in person-centred care through enabling of nurses to transform the culture and context of care... it is enabled and supported by facilitators committed to a systematic, rigorous and continuous process of emancipatory change (McCormack et al 1999:256).

Nomenclature used in the literature to describe the concept of Practice Development is confusing. In the 1960s, there was the pioneering concept in the US of the 'Care, Core and Cure' model (Hall 1966). From this early concept, came the 1980s UK model of 'Nursing Development Units' initiated by Alan Pearson (Malby 1996, Salvage 1995). In Australia, the concept emerged as 'Clinical Development Units, Nursing' (Greenwood 1999). The concept continued evolving in the UK to the 1990s model of 'Practice Development Units' (McCormack et al 1999). The change in nomenclature is accompanied by slight variations in the philosophy and focus of the concept of Practice Development. Regardless of the nomenclature used to label Practice Development, key components consistent with most descriptions of the concept include:

- responding to identified patients' needs
- improving services to patients
- utilising evidence to support practice
- improving the effectiveness of the service
- improving the professional's role, knowledge and/or skills, and
- empowering nurses to introduce change to improve practice (Greenwood 1999, McCormack & Garbett 2003, Pearson 1989, Salvage 1995, Unsworth 2000).

More recently, the importance of facilitation in ensuring the success of Practice Development has been advocated. A trained and experienced facilitator committed to enabling nurses to critically interrogate their practice, using an evidence-based approach towards efficient and effective practice change through research, is key (McCormack & Garbett 2003, McCormack et al 1999, Thompson et al 2001, Unsworth 2000). Clinically credible nurses within the practice environment, such as clinical nurse specialists, clinical educators and Practice Development nurses, provide the most effective route to enabling nurses to use research in practice (Thompson et al 2001). Practice Development methodology brings together, under the guidance of these trained and experienced facilitators, the simultaneous development of the nurse while improving outcomes for the patient using an EBP approach.

Although there is a plethora of literature on the nature and benefits of Practice Development (Greenwood 2000, Greenwood 1999, Kitson et al 1996, Manley & McCormack 2003, McCormack et al 1999, McCormack & Garbett 2003, Unsworth 2000), the term remains nebulous with clinicians (Clarke & Proctor 1999, Tolson 1999). In addition, there is little published literature systematically evaluating a Practice Development methodology in the Australian or international context (Draper 1996, Gerrish 2001, Osborne 2009). However, with its 'bottom-up' approach and theoretical underpinnings of critical social science theory, the central aim of Practice Development remains to develop a culture of inquiry.

3.8 Conclusion

This chapter has explored the concepts of EBP and culture. We have also conceptualised what is meant by an 'evidence-based culture' and discussed in detail ways in which the organisation and the individual nurse can work together to achieve this 'culture of inquiry'. Without the requisite infrastructure, resources, support, opportunities and incentives necessary to enable evidence-based nursing practice, as well as to enable the generation of nurse-initiated evidence for practice through the conduct of research, it will not be possible for organisations to sustain the transformation into a culture of inquiry.

3.9 DISCUSSION QUESTIONS

1. What are some of the characteristics of a culture of inquiry? Which of these characteristics are evident in your organisation?
2. What are some strategies for developing a culture of inquiry? What strategies could be used in your organisation?
3. Compare the Magnet Hospital concept with the Practice Development concept in relation to building a culture of inquiry. Consider which characteristics of each would suit your organisation's strategic plan for cultural change.

3.10 References

Aiken L H, Sloane D M, Lake E 1994 Lower Medicare mortality among a set of hospitals known for good nursing care. *Medical Care* 32(8):771–87.

Aiken L H, Sloane D M, Lake E 1997 Satisfaction with inpatient AIDS care: a national comparison of dedicated and scattered-bed units. *Medical Care* 35(9):948–62.

Aiken L H, Sloane D M, Lake E T et al 1999 Organization and outcomes of inpatient AIDS care. *Medical Care* 37(8):760–72.

American Nurses Credentialing Center (ANCC) 2003 *ANCC Magnet Program: recognizing excellence in nursing services.* Available: www.nursingworld.org/default.aspx 8 May 2009.

Baggs J G, Schmitt M H, Mushlin A I et al 1999 Association between nurse–physician collaboration and patient outcomes in three intensive care units. *Critical Care Medicine* 27(9):1991–8.

Ballou K A 1998 A concept analysis of autonomy. *Journal of Professional Nursing* 14(2):102–10.

Bate P 1994 *Strategies for cultural change.* Butterworth-Heinemann, Oxford.

Blanchfield K C, Biordi D L 1996 Power in practice: a study of nursing authority and autonomy. *Nursing Administration Quarterly* 20(3):42–9.

Bland C J, Ruffin M T 1992 Characteristics of a productive research environment: literature review. *Academic Medicine* 67(6):385–97.

Brown C E, Wickline M A, Ecoff I et al 2009 Nursing practice, knowledge, attitudes and perceived barriers to evidence-based practice at an academic medical center. *Journal of Advanced Nursing* 65(2):371–81.

Bryar R M, Closs S J, Baum G et al 2003 The Yorkshire BARRIERS project: diagnostic analysis of barriers to research utilisation. *International Journal of Nursing Studies* 40(1):73–84.

Carlson C L, Plonczynski D J 2008 Has the BARRIERS scale changed nursing practice? An integrative review. *Journal of Advanced Nursing* 63(4):322–33.

Clarke C, Proctor S 1999 Practice development: ambiguity in research and practice. *Journal of Advanced Nursing* 30(4):975–82.

Draper J 1996 Nursing development units: an opportunity for evaluation. *Journal of Advanced Nursing* 23(2):267–71.

Fay B 1987 *Critical social science.* Cornell University Press, Ithaca, NY.

Fink R, Thompson C J, Bonnes D 2005 Overcoming barriers and promoting the use of research in practice. *Journal of Nursing Administration* 35(3):121–9.

Forbes A, Griffiths P 2002 Methodological strategies for the identification and synthesis of 'evidence' to support decision-making in relation to complex healthcare systems and practices. *Nursing Inquiry* 9(3):141–55.

Foxcroft D R, Cole N, Fulbrook P 2000 (updated 2009) Organisational infrastructures to promote evidence-based nursing practice. *Cochrane Database of Systematic Reviews*, Issue 3. Art no: CD002212. DOI: 10.1002/14651858.CD002212.

Funk S G, Champagne M T, Wiese R A et al 1991 Barriers to using research findings in practice: the clinician's perspective *Applied Nursing Research*. 4(2):90–5.

Gerrish K 2001 A pluralistic evaluation of nursing/practice development units. *Journal of Clinical Nursing* 10(1):109–18.

Greenhalgh T, Robert G, MacFarlane F et al 2004 Diffusion of innovations in service organizations: systematic review and recommendations. *Milbank Quarterly* 82(4): 581–629.

Greenwood J 1999 Clinical development units (nursing): the Western Sydney approach. *Journal of Advanced Nursing* 29(3):674–9.

Greenwood J 2000 Clinical development units (nursing): issues surrounding their establishment and survival. *International Journal of Nursing Practice* 6:338–44.

Hall L E 1966 Another view of nursing care and quality. In: Straub M, Parker K (eds) *Continuity of patient care: the role of nursing*. Catholic University of America Press, Washington, DC.

Havens D S 2001 Comparing nursing infrastructure and outcomes: ANCC magnet and nonmagnet CNEs report. *Nursing Economics* 19:258–66.

Havens D S, Aiken L H 1999 Shaping systems to promote desired outcomes: the Magnet Hospital model. *Journal of Nursing Administration* 29(2):14–20.

Havens D, Vasey J 2003 Measuring staff nurse decisional involvement. The decisional involvement scale. *Journal of Nursing Administration* 33(6):331–6.

Heater B S, Becker A M, Olson R K 1988 Nursing interventions and patient outcomes: a meta-analysis of studies. *Nursing Research* 37(5):303–7.

Hesselbein F 2002 The key to cultural transformation. In: Hesselbein F, Johnston R (eds) *On leading change: a leader to leader guide*. Jossey-Bass, Indianapolis, IN.

Holland C K 1993 An ethnographic study of nursing culture as an exploration for determining the existence of a system of ritual. *Journal of Advanced Nursing* 18(9):1461–70.

Kajermo K N, Nordstrom G, Krusebrant A et al 1998 Barriers to and facilitators of research utilization, as perceived by a group of registered nurses in Sweden. *Journal of Advanced Nursing* 27:798–807.

Kitson A, Ahmed L B, Harvey G et al 1996 From research to practice: one organizational model for promoting research-based practice. *Journal of Advanced Nursing* 23(3):430–40.

Kitson A, Harvey G, McCormack B 1998 Enabling the implementation of evidence-based practice: a conceptual framework. *Journal of Professional Nursing* 21(6):335–44.

Kramer M, Schmalenberg C E 2003a Magnet Hospital nurses describe control over nursing practice. *Western Journal of Nursing Research* 25(4):434–52.

Kramer M, Schmalenberg C E 2003b Magnet Hospital staff nurses describe clinical autonomy. *Nursing Outlook* 51(1):13–19.

Kramer M, Schmalenberg C 2005 Best quality patient care: a historical perspective on Magnet Hospitals. *Nursing Administration Quarterly* 29(3):275–87.

Malby R 1996 Nursing development units in the United Kingdom. *Advanced Practice Nursing Quarterly* 1(4):20–7.

Manley K, McCormack B 2003 Practice development: purpose, methodology, facilitation and evaluation. *Nursing in Critical Care* 8:22–9.

McClure M, Poulin M, Sovie M D 1983 *Magnet Hospitals: attraction and retention of professional nurses*. American Academy of Nurses, American Nurses Association, Kansas City, MO.

McCormack B, Garbett R 2003 The characteristics, qualities and skills of practice developers. *Journal of Clinical Nursing* 12(3):317–25.

McCormack B, Manley K, Kitson A et al 1999 Towards practice development: a vision in reality or a reality without vision? *Journal of Nursing Management* 7(5):255–64.

Miller J R, Messenger S R 1978 Obstacles to applying nursing research findings. *American Journal of Nursing* 78(4):632–4.

Newhouse R P, Dearholt S, Poe S et al 2005 Evidence-based practice: a practical approach to implementation. *Journal of Nursing Administration* 35(1):35–40.

Newhouse R P 2007 Creating infrastructure supportive of evidence-based nursing practice: leadership strategies. *Worldviews on Evidence-Based Nursing* 4(1):21–9.

O'Callaghan J 2001 Do rituals still rule over research evidence? *Australian Nursing Journal* 8(8):39–40.

Osborne S 2009 Testing the effectiveness of a nursing practice development intervention on changing the culture of evidence-based practice in an acute care environment. PhD thesis. Queensland University of Technology, Queensland.

Osborne S R, Gardner G 2004 Imperatives and strategies for developing an evidence-based practice in perioperative nursing. *ACORN Journal* 17(1):18–24.

Parahoo K, McCaughan E M 2001 Research utilization among medical and surgical nurses: a comparison of their self reports and perceptions of barriers and facilitators. *Journal of Nursing Management* 9(1):21–30.

Pearson A 1989 Therapeutic nursing: transforming models and theories in action. *Recent Advances in Nursing* 24:123–51.

Retsas A 2000 Barriers to using research evidence in nursing practice. *Journal of Advanced Nursing* 31:599–606.

Rosswurm M A, Larrabee J H 1999 A model for change to evidence-based practice. *Image: Journal of Nursing Scholarship* 31(4):317–22.

Rycroft-Malone J 2004 The PARIHS framework: a framework for guiding the implementation of evidence-based practice. *Journal of Nursing Care Quality* 19(4):297–304.

Salvage J 1995 Greenhouses, flagships and umbrellas. In: Salvage J, Wright S G (eds) *Nursing development units: a force for change.* Scutari Press, London.

Schein E H 1992 *Organizational culture and leadership, 2nd edn.* Jossey-Bass, San Francisco, CA.

Scott J G, Sochalski J, Aiken L H 1999 Review of Magnet Hospital research: findings and implications for professional nursing practice. *Journal of Nursing Administration* 29(1):9–19.

Stetler C B 2001 Updating the Stetler model of research utilization to facilitate evidence-based practice. *Nursing Outlook* 49(6):272–9.

Stevens K R 2004 *ACE star model of EBP: knowledge transformation.* Academic Center for Evidence-Based Practice, The University of Texas Health Science Center, San Antonio, TX.

Titler M G, Kleiber C, Steelman V J et al 2001 The Iowa Model of evidence-based practice to promote quality care. *Critical Care Nursing Clinics of North America* 13(4):497–509.

Stolzenberger K M 2003 Beyond the Magnet award: the ANCC Magnet program as the framework for culture change. *Journal of Nursing Administration* 33(10):522–31.

Strange F 2002 The persistence of ritual in nursing practice. *Clinical Effectiveness in Nursing* 5(4):177–83.

Thiel L, Ghosh Y 2008 Determining registered nurses' readiness for evidence-based practice. *Worldviews on Evidence-Based Nursing* 5(4):182–92.

Thompson C, McCaughan D, Cullum N et al 2001 The accessibility of research-based knowledge for nurses in United Kingdom acute care settings. *Journal of Advanced Nursing* 36(1):11–22.

Tolson D 1999 Practice innovation: a methodological maze. *Journal of Advanced Nursing* 30(2):381–90.

Tranmer J E, Coulson K, Holtom D et al 1998 The emergence of a culture that promotes evidence-based clinical decision making within an acute care setting. *Canadian Journal of Nursing Administration* 11(2):36–58.

Turkel M C, Reidinger G, Ferket K et al 2005 An essential component of the magnet journey: fostering an environment for evidence-based practice and nursing research. *Nursing Administration Quarterly* 29(3):254–62.

Unsworth J 2000 Practice development: a concept analysis. *Journal of Nursing Management* 8(6):317–26.

Webb S S, Price S A, Van Ess Coeling H 1996 Valuing authority/responsibility relationships: the essence of professional practice. *Journal of Nursing Administration* 26:28–33.

Winslow E H 1998 Questioning the chains of habit. *Journal of Cardiovascular Nursing* 12(2):94–108.

CHAPTER **4**

Development and use of clinical guidelines

Sonya Osborne and Joan Webster

4.1 Learning objectives

After reading this chapter, you should be able to:
1. identify the key criteria and characteristics of effective clinical guidelines
2. discuss the benefits and limitations of evidence-based guidelines
3. apply a conceptual framework in the guideline development processes, and
4. apply key principles in the implementation, and evaluation, of evidence-based guidelines into practice.

4.2 Introduction

The purpose of this chapter is to provide an overview of the development and use of clinical guidelines as a tool for decision making in clinical practice. Nurses have always developed and used tools to guide clinical decision making related to interventions in practice. Since Florence Nightingale (Nightingale 1860) gave us 'notes' on nursing in the late 1800s, nurses have continued to use tools, such as standards, policies and procedures, protocols, algorithms, clinical pathways and clinical guidelines, to assist them in making appropriate decisions about patient care that eventuate in the best desired patient outcomes.

Clinical guidelines have enjoyed growing popularity as a comprehensive tool for synthesising clinical evidence and information into user-friendly recommendations for practice. Historically, clinical guidelines were developed by individual experts or groups of experts by consensus, with no transparent process for the user to determine the validity and reliability of the recommendations. The acceptance of the evidence-based practice (EBP) movement as a paradigm for clinical decision making underscores the imperative for clinical guidelines to be systematically developed and based on the best available research evidence.

Clinicians are faced with the dilemma of choosing from an abundance of guidelines of variable quality, or developing new guidelines. Where do you start? How do you find an existing guideline to fit your practice? How do you know if a guideline is evidence-based, valid and reliable? Should you apply an existing guideline in your practice or develop a new guideline? How do you get clinicians to use the guidelines? How do you know if using the guideline will make any difference in care delivery or patient outcomes? Whatever the choice, the challenge lies in choosing or developing a clinical guideline that is credible as a decision-making tool for the delivery of quality, efficient and effective care. This chapter will address the posed questions through an exploration of the ins and outs of clinical guidelines, from development to application to evaluation.

4.3 What are clinical guidelines?

Before getting into this chapter on clinical guidelines, it is necessary to start with a definition to differentiate clinical guidelines from the myriad of other decision-making tools nurses use in practice (see Table 4.1). However, it is important to keep in mind that regardless of nomenclature (e.g. algorithm, clinical pathway), the process of the development of clinical decision-making tools should be equally as rigorous. Clinical guidelines are 'systematically developed statements to assist practitioner and patient decisions about appropriate healthcare for specific circumstances' (Field & Lohr 1992). The broad purpose of clinical guidelines is to aid clinicians in providing quality care and to aid in the evaluation of that care against best practice.

Evidence-based guidelines have been promoted as one strategy for bridging the research–practice gap by translating research findings into feasible recommendations ready for integration into practice. The proliferation of guidelines in the past 15 years has been an attempt to address the problems of variability in practice and inappropriate practice, by gathering together in one place the best available evidence to support effective and efficient care. There is some evidence that guideline-driven care by medical, nursing and allied health professionals can be effective, in varying degrees, in changing the process and improving the outcome of care (Grimshaw & Russell 1993, Thomas et al 2003).

However, in order for guidelines to reach their full potential, they must be: developed with the end user in mind; developed using systematic and rigorous processes; developed simultaneously with dissemination and implementation strategies; and evaluated regularly

---

Algorithms are clinical guidelines prepared in a flowchart format. They typically describe the process and decisions, allow for alternative pathways and are involved in addressing a specific condition.

Clinical pathways are typically multidisciplinary management tools based on clinical information developed in other guidelines. They document the essential steps in a clinical process from hospital admission to discharge, detailing the timing of interventions to achieve identified outcomes.

Clinical guidelines are systematically developed statements to assist clinical and patient decisions about appropriate healthcare for specific clinical circumstances (Field & Lohr 1992).

Policies are written plans of an organisation's official position, based on the organisation's purpose and goals, on a specific health situation. They are intended to guide and determine decisions for improving a specific health situation.

Procedures are an established series of ordered steps for performing specific tasks, typically associated with an identified policy.

Protocols are rigid, prescribed statements. They describe in detail how the process of the most cost-effective care for a population of patients should be conducted, usually to expedite care for routine problems.

Standards are accepted discipline-based principles for patient care processes, developed to increase the probability of appropriate care.

Table 4.1 Examples of clinical decision-making tools used in practice

to keep abreast of the ever-changing healthcare environment and new knowledge. With this in mind, clinicians must be aware that not all guidelines have been developed within the confines of the above criteria or without the impact of other influences inherent in the current processes. Some of the issues that can cloud the credibility and acceptance of a guideline as evidence-based include: conflicting or lack of research evidence; governance and composition of the guideline development committee; unanimity among committee stakeholders within the development process; lack of transparency in the consensus process; lack of independent external review; resource availability or constraints; and conflict of interests among stakeholders, industry and academia (Raine et al 2005, Sniderman & Furberg 2009). Guidelines must be critically appraised before they are accepted for use in practice; only then can guidelines effectively assist in clinical decision making, improve the quality of healthcare, guide resource allocation and reduce the legal risk of liability.

4.4 What are the characteristics of effective clinical guidelines?

Grilli et al (2000) evaluated 431 guidelines produced by professional specialty organisations between 1988 and 1998 for quality, based on three dimensions: description of stakeholder involvement in the development process; strategy for identifying evidence; and grading of recommendations. Only 5% of guidelines in the study met all three criteria for quality, which led to the conclusion that 'explicit methodological criteria for the production of guidelines shared among public agencies, scientific societies, and patients' associations need to be set up' (Grilli et al 2000:103).

Although there is no internationally recognised and universally accepted framework for the development of clinical guidelines, guideline development organisations around the world are in agreement on certain key qualities required for guidelines to be effective. These key qualities include validity, reproducibility, representativeness, flexibility, adaptability, cost-effectiveness, applicability, reliability and usefulness (Field & Lohr 1992; NHMRC 1999, 2009; SIGN 2001). These key qualities should be considered when appraising existing national clinical guidelines before adaptation to local contexts, and when developing new guidelines. Guideline development methodology, and therefore guidelines, can be enhanced worldwide by the adoption of an internationally accepted conceptual framework, based on the recognised key qualities. In this way, internationally accepted standards for the collection and synthesis of evidence in developing effective guidelines can be established.

More recently, the World Health Organisation (WHO) commissioned a series of 16 reviews to address the need to use more rigorous processes for guideline development (Oxman et al 2006). Schünemann et al (2006) found no experimental research that compared the different components of guidelines. They did find many examples, surveys and other observational studies that compared the impact of different guideline development documents on guideline quality, and recommended integration of key components similar to those recommended by the National Health and Medical Research Council (NHMRC) in the late 1990s (NHMRC 1999).

In Australia, the NHMRC (1999, 2009) has incorporated recognised key qualities into nine guiding principles for effective guideline development. These nine principles have been adapted and presented as a conceptual framework for guideline development in Table 4.2.

4.4.1 Principle 1: guideline development should be outcome-focused

Guidelines should be developed with inferences about specific clinical and economic outcomes. The validity of the guideline can then be assessed on how implementation of the recommendations compares with alternative treatment or management in achieving the projected outcomes.

Key qualities	Guideline development principles
Valid and reproducible	Guideline development should be outcome-focused.
	Guidelines should be based on best available evidence and describe the strength of the link between recommendation and outcome.
	Guideline evidence should be combined using the strongest method available to determine effect on clinical outcomes.
Representative	Guideline development teams should be multidisciplinary and include consumer representatives.
Flexible and adaptable	Guidelines should be flexible and adaptable to local conditions.
Cost-effective	Guidelines should be developed with thought to resource limits.
Reliable and applicable	Guidelines should be developed with thought to the target audience.
	Guidelines should be evaluated for effect, value, validity and usage.
	Guidelines should be reviewed and modified regularly to incorporate new evidence.

Table 4.2 Conceptual framework for guideline development
Source: Adapted from NHMRC's nine guiding principles underlying the guideline development process (NHMRC 1999)

4.4.2 Principle 2: guidelines should be based on best available evidence and describe the strength of the link between recommendation and outcome

Searching for and analysing research evidence is the most expensive and time-consuming component of evidence-based guideline development (Browman 2001), and may sometimes be an impetus for taking shortcuts in the process. Meticulous processes must be adhered to so that the credibility and validity of the guideline is assured. Systematic reviews, including a meta-analysis of results, are accepted by researchers as being at the top of the hierarchy of evidence pyramid. Despite this, a review of the use of systematic reviews in clinical guidelines found that only 3% of the references cited were systematic reviews (Grant et al 2000). The authority of systematic reviews of the literature depends a great deal on the care of the search conducted (Grilli et al 2000). Furthermore, conventionally, the gold standard of experimental research is a randomised controlled design, because randomisation strengthens the internal validity of the design and the findings. However, a randomised controlled design is not always appropriate or feasible in clinical practice when evaluating the effectiveness of complex interventions on change, in situations where contextual factors cannot be controlled and the nature of the intervention does not lend itself to standardisation (Osborne 2009). Thus, not all guideline recommendations can be underpinned by systematic reviews, and guideline developers can and should make recommendations that are specific to local contexts.

In addition to a careful search for evidence, the grading of that evidence is essential to discriminate evidence-based from consensus-based recommendations (Grilli et al 2000). The effectiveness of guidelines depends on the quality of the evidence upon which they are based. Guidelines should be accompanied by explicit details on how the research was judged for level of evidence, methodological quality, relevance to the research question and applicability to the target patient population. A guide to grading the recommendations based on the strength of the link between the evidence and the recommendation should be made evident.

4.4.3 Principle 3: guideline evidence should be combined using the strongest method available to determine effect on clinical outcomes

Good quality evidence is necessary but not enough when making recommendations (NHMRC 1999). The availability of evidence from one high-level study does not immediately mean a good clinical recommendation will result, due to issues such as small effect size or the use of non-clinical outcomes (NHMRC 1999). In addition, one of the difficulties in searching the literature is determining effect size where there is conflicting evidence. Where more than one study is available, appropriate combination of results into a meta-analysis may yield a truer picture of treatment effect. The guideline development team must be able to assess and combine not only the effect of interventions, but also the feasibility of implementation relevant to resources, and inequities that may arise in certain populations gaining access to the recommended treatment (NHMRC 1999).

4.4.4 Principle 4: guideline development teams should be multidisciplinary and include consumer representatives

Guideline development teams should be diverse and representative of all stakeholders (e.g. medical officers, nurses, allied health professionals, consumers, policy makers, health facility managers and pharmacists). A representative team can engage in a more holistic discussion of all aspects of a topic, such as relevant outcomes, patient values and barriers to implementation, instead of writing the guideline from one perspective. Involvement of all relevant stakeholders will improve the quality and continuity of care, and improve the likelihood of uptake of guideline recommendations by all (NHMRC 1999). Care must be taken in assembling the guideline development team and systems should be in place so that all team members have adequate input into the decision-making processes.

4.4.5 Principle 5: guidelines should be flexible and adaptable to local conditions

Local adaptation of existing guidelines is necessary to ensure the guidelines meet the issues of quality, validity and applicability in the immediate setting. The NHMRC recommends that national guidelines must be flexible and amenable to local adaptation by:
- providing evidence of relevance to different target populations, different geographic settings and different clinic settings
- considering resource implications, including costs and benefits, and
- providing a way to incorporate patient values and preferences (NHMRC 1999).

4.4.6 Principle 6: guidelines should be developed with thought to resource limits

Clinical guidelines should be mindful of resource implications and provide an economic analysis of consequences if the guideline recommendations are used and if they are not used. When adapting guidelines for the local setting, consideration should be given to several factors, including alternative treatment options, availability of equipment, variability in education, knowledge and skill, and availability of clinicians to follow through on the recommendations (NHMRC 1999). Knowledge of the economic analyses will be useful in the clinicians' decision-making process of whether to follow the guideline recommendations or choose an alternative course of action, depending on the above-mentioned factors.

4.4.7 Principle 7: guidelines should be developed with thought to the target audience

The target audience or end users of the guideline should be considered when developing strategies to disseminate and implement guideline recommendations. The target audience includes not only clinicians who will be involved in implementation of care recommendations, but also patients who will be recipients of that care. Guidelines are only as effective as their awareness, understanding and use in practice allow. The guideline must be introduced to the target audience through targeted dissemination and education strategies in conjunction with proactive strategies for overcoming barriers to uptake and use.

4.4.8 Principle 8: guidelines should be evaluated for effect, value, validity and usage

Clinical effectiveness of guidelines depends on resolution of identified problems that are the focus of the guideline. Therefore, health outcomes must be monitored after guideline implementation to determine the impact of the guideline. The impact of the guideline on clinician knowledge and practice behaviour must also be evaluated to obtain a clearer picture of the use of the guideline in practice. It is important that the guideline be evaluated for perceptions of relevance and importance to clinicians and patients, as this will have an impact on compliance with guideline recommendations.

4.4.9 Principle 9: guidelines should be reviewed and modified regularly to incorporate new evidence

Clinical guidelines become obsolete in the face of new evidence and must therefore be regularly reviewed and modified. Using the evidence-based approach to guideline development creates a solid foundation for subsequent review because any subsequent review should not have to be entirely redone, but updated from the point of the last review (Browman 2001). Shekelle et al (2001) estimate that the average 'life span' of a guideline is 3 years; however, more frequent updates using rigorous methods may be easier to accomplish and more valid than infrequent updates that compromise rigour to make up for lost time (Browman 2001).

4.5 How should clinical guidelines be used in practice?

The purpose of evidence-based guidelines is to assist practitioners in providing quality care by serving as a useful aid for clinical decision making (Field & Lohr 1992). The use of guidelines in conjunction with clinician expertise and judgment, as well as knowledge of the patient, enables clinicians to make decisions that incorporate best practice into individual patient care. Guidelines are useful in assessing and assuring the quality of care (Field & Lohr 1992), and establishing best practice (Keogh & Courtney 2001). Evaluation of quality of care is enhanced by using the guideline as a framework for comparison of current practice with best practice. In this way, guidelines may also be useful in reducing risk of legal liability or negligence (Field & Lohr 1992), by establishing standards for best practice that a reasonable clinician would follow in light of the evidence available.

Guidelines are also useful in the allocation of resources and reduction of healthcare costs (Field & Lohr 1992, Keogh & Courtney 2001). Guidelines can identify recommendations for appropriate and cost-effective management of clinical conditions. Guidelines are also useful in streamlining processes (Keogh & Courtney 2001), which contributes to the best use of available resources. So, how do you use these evidence-based guidelines for practice?

4.5.1 Finding existing guidelines

Clinical guidelines can readily be found in print and electronic form, although a wider search can be made electronically via the internet. Electronically searching for clinical guidelines may involve a variety of resources. These include general guideline database archives (e.g. US National Guideline Clearinghouse); specialty guideline database archives (e.g. Royal College of Nursing clinical guidelines site); citation databases (e.g. CINAHL®, MEDLINE® and EMBASE); and internet search engines (e.g. Google). General and specialty-specific guideline archive databases are produced and maintained by hundreds of organisations around the world. A brief list of guideline development organisations can be found in Table 4.3. Internet search engines are also numerous and differ in their strategies for searching, the options available and the coverage offered (McSweeney et al 2001). Using a combination of the above resources will result in a considerable amount of information; therefore, a targeted search strategy and quality filtering strategy will increase the chances of retrieving only relevant and useful guidelines.

To put the quantity of clinical guidelines in perspective, a recent electronic search of MEDLINE, CINAHL and the Cochrane Library using the search term 'guideline' resulted in 79,044 hits, up from 6218 hits in 2004. Similarly, a search on the search engine Google using the term 'clinical guideline' resulted in 34,200,000 hits, up from 360,000 hits obtained just 5 years ago. The potential amount of information available should serve as an imperative for having a strategy for quickly evaluating the context and content of the guideline. In other words, how can you assess the quality of a guideline?

4.5.2 Appraising existing guidelines

The availability of an existing guideline does not guarantee its quality, validity or applicability. Several specialty organisations may produce guidelines for the same clinical issue but offer different recommendations for practice. Whose recommendations should

Resource	Country of origin	Available:
National Health and Medical Research Council (NHMRC)	Australia	www.nhmrc.gov.au/publications/synopses/cp30syn.htm
National Health Service National Institute for Health and Clinical Excellence (NICE)	UK	www.nice.org.uk
Agency for Healthcare Research and Quality (AHRQ)	USA	www.ahrq.gov
Canadian Medical Association (CMA)	Canada	www.cma.ca/index.cfm/ci_id/121/la_id/1.htm
Guidelines International Network (GIN)	International	www.g-i-n.net/guidelines
Joanna Briggs Institute (JBI)	Australia	www.joannabriggs.edu.au/about/home.php
New Zealand Guidelines Group (NZGG)	New Zealand	www.nzgg.org.nz
Registered Nurses' Association of Ontario	Canada	www.rnao.org
Royal College of Nursing (RCN)	UK	www.rcn.org.uk
Scottish Intercollegiate Guidelines Network (SIGN)	UK	www.sign.ac.uk/index.html
National Guideline Clearinghouse	USA	www.guideline.gov

Table 4.3 Guideline resources

you follow, if any? Just as principles have been described for developing guidelines, similar principles must be used in evaluating the quality of existing guidelines. Fortunately, the principles of guideline development can also be applied to guideline evaluation.

Several critical appraisal evaluation checklists are available to help in considering application of a guideline in practice (Hayward et al 1995a, 1995b; AGREE Collaboration 2001). One example of a guideline appraisal checklist is the Appraisal of Guidelines, Research and Evaluation (AGREE) instrument, a generic guideline appraisal checklist (AGREE Collaboration 2001). The AGREE instrument is a user-friendly tool that focuses on six domains: scope and purpose; stakeholder involvement; rigour of development; clarity and presentation; applicability; and editorial independence. The AGREE domains can be superimposed upon the previously presented conceptual framework for guideline development to demonstrate that the same criteria for developing guidelines can and should be used to evaluate guidelines for use.

In light of the amount of information you may find through an electronic search, there must be a way to 'weed out' more useful and relevant guidelines for retrieval and further assessment. Three simple questions, which are the basis of most appraisal checklists (Ciliska et al 2001; Hayward et al 1995a, 1995b; McSweeney et al 2001), can be asked: What are the recommendations? Are the recommendations valid? Will the recommendations help me in caring for my patients?

> Busy clinicians might hope that criteria for appraising practice guidelines
> would obviate the need for reviewing how the guideline developers have
> brought together the evidence, and how they have chosen the values reflected
> in their recommendations. Unfortunately, any shortcuts that bypass at least
> a cursory look at evidence and values will leave the clinician open to being
> misled by guidelines that may be based on a biased selection of evidence,
> a skewed interpretation of that evidence, or an idiosyncratic set of values
> (Hayward et al 1995a:571).

A word of caution… in appraising guidelines for quality, validity and applicability, attention must be given to the fact that guideline recommendations are influenced by the values of the organisation producing the guideline, in relation to the objective of having an effect on how clinicians practice. So, how do you decide whether to adapt an existing guideline or develop a new one?

4.5.3 Adapting existing guidelines for local use or developing new guidelines

Guideline development can be a costly, resource-intensive and time-consuming undertaking. It may better suit the needs of the organisation, team or individual to make use of the work of others, particularly national guideline development bodies and specialty organisations, instead of 'reinventing the wheel'. There are advantages and disadvantages to both approaches, although the most resource-sparing venture is to adapt existing guidelines. Regardless of the approach taken, whether adapted from national guidelines or developed locally, uptake of evidence-based guidelines is enhanced if the guideline is disseminated in user-friendly formats such as algorithms, clinical pathways, policies and procedures, standards or protocols for practice.

The main disadvantages of developing guidelines from scratch are the large investment in resources, the time constraints that may negatively affect the process, and the need to hire or train clinicians in guideline development processes, small group leadership and facilitation, and information management. However, the advantages of developing guidelines at the local level include capacity building in EBP, and improved uptake, use and evaluation of the guideline recommendations because of a cultural sense of 'ownership'.

As mentioned previously, local adaptation of existing guidelines is necessary to ensure the guidelines meet quality, validity and applicability issues in the immediate setting. When adapting existing guidelines, the starting point should be a high-quality guideline. The existing guideline should have the same focus as the topic of local need and the guideline should be assessed using the same conceptual framework for developing a guideline. So, what is involved in the process of developing clinical guidelines?

4.6 How are guidelines developed?

The quality of the guideline development process influences the likely use of the guidelines in practice. The way in which guidelines are developed strongly influences their acceptance and the extent to which they are subsequently used (Field & Lohr 1992, Grimshaw et al 1995, Pagliari & Grimshaw 2002). There is international consensus by national guideline development agencies that the principles of EBP influence the development of guidelines (Burgers et al 2003). Steps in guideline development thus mimic steps in the EBP process (see Ch 1 for a review of the EBP process). These steps include: selection and focus of the topic; systematic search for scientific evidence; critical review and synthesis of best evidence into recommendations; application and implementation of the guideline in practice; and evaluation of the guideline for compliance, efficiency and effectiveness. Each of these steps will be explained in more detail below, and the process is summarised in Figure 4.1.

4.6.1 Selection and focus of the topic

Before embarking on the resource-intensive journey of developing a clinical practice guideline, the topic is selected and focused, and the project scoped. There is usually local *anecdotal* evidence of the need for a guideline on a particular topic to address variability in practice and improve patient outcomes.

Some preliminary work must be conducted to determine whether there is *authentic* evidence to support the need. Topics are amenable to guidelines if there is uncertainty about appropriate practice, if there is variation in practice among clinicians, and if there are significant cost benefits in changing practice, without sacrificing effectiveness (Webster et al 1999).

The guideline topic can be focused using the same methods for formulating clinical questions in the EBP process (see Ch 1), whereby the patient or population with a specific health condition, as well as measurable health outcomes, are identified.

It is well-recognised and accepted that guidelines should be developed by multidisciplinary groups and based on systematic review of the scientific evidence; and that recommendations should be clearly linked to the supporting evidence and graded according to the strength of that evidence (Harbour & Miller 2001). Once this preliminary work is complete, a guideline development team must be established to progress the project. Ideally, this multidisciplinary team should be comprised of representatives from all stakeholder groups, such as nursing, medicine and allied health, and especially a patient or consumer representative. Another valuable member of the team is a health science librarian and at least one member trained and experienced in the critical appraisal of research.

One of the first responsibilities of the guideline development team is to come to an agreement on the purpose of the guideline, the end users or target audience, the context of guideline use, the condition or problem of focus, and the measurable outcomes that

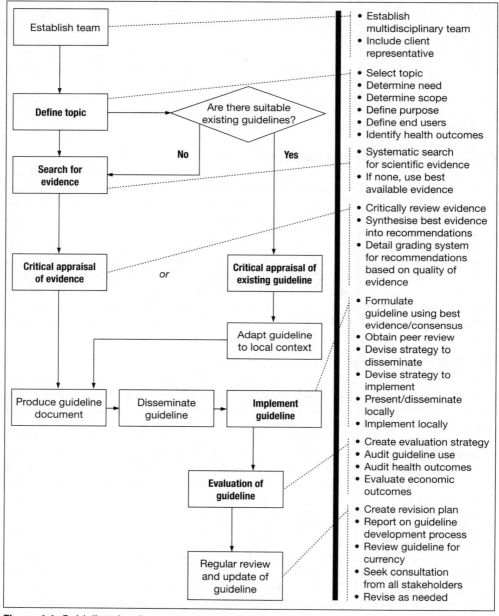

Figure 4.1 Guideline development process

the guideline will address. A health outcome is a change in health status as a result of the appropriate choice of interventions by the healthcare provider (Donabedian 1992, NHMRC 1999). Examples of outcome measures recognised by the NHMRC include general health status, early or late morbidity, treatment complications, mortality, relapse or readmission rates, complication rates, return to work, physical and social functioning, quality of life and patient satisfaction (NHMRC 1999).

It is important for the guideline development team to be clear about the focus of the guideline, especially the problem and the outcomes, as this will not only serve as the basis for evaluation down the track, but will immediately inform and guide the search for evidence.

4.6.2 Systematically search for scientific evidence

In order to ensure that the guideline is based on the best research evidence available, a systematic search of the literature is conducted. A properly conducted and reported systematic review creates a solid foundation for recommendations that are as current as they are practical (Browman 2001). Formulation of a comprehensive search strategy, using the relevant terms, is the first step in conducting a systematic search. The second step is searching the relevant literature, which includes searching electronic databases such as CINAHL, MEDLINE and EMBASE, hand-searching relevant journals, searching proceedings from relevant conferences, and consulting with any other professional organisations or experts in the field who may be aware of unpublished research. The search strategy is defined not only by the patient group and outcomes under consideration, but also by the type of study design used to answer the question.

Guidelines typically are concerned with best treatment or intervention alternatives. Therefore, using a hierarchical ranking of the quality of research for intervention studies, a systematic review with meta-analysis of all randomised controlled trials (RCTs) is at the top of the evidence pyramid, followed by a well-conducted RCT. In the absence of RCTs for intervention studies, other types of evidence from other study designs may be used to guide recommendations (see Ch 2 for a review of types of evidence and types of study designs).

Several guideline development organisations have suggested the use of an evidence table or balance sheet to manage the evidence collection process (NHMRC 1999, SIGN 2001). An example of an evidence table can be found on the Scottish Intercollegiate Guidelines Network (SIGN) website (see www.sign.ac.uk/index.html). In the absence of available research studies, expert opinion and consensus are other sources of evidence, albeit not as strong as evidence obtained from well-designed research studies. In any case, a transparent process for ranking the evidence based on type of study design, quality of study evidence, and strength of recommendation should be made explicit in the guideline. Credibility of the guideline recommendations depends on the quality of the evidence and the explicit link between the research evidence and the recommendations.

4.6.3 Critically review and synthesise best evidence into recommendations

Once the evidence is gathered, the next task is to critically appraise the evidence and synthesise the best evidence into recommendations. Well-constructed guideline documents contain explicit descriptions about the level of evidence used as support, how the quality of the evidence was determined, and how the strength of the recommendation was established. The level of evidence is based on the study design (e.g. an RCT). The quality of the evidence is based on the appropriateness of the study design to answer the study question and the validity of the findings. The key to critical appraisal is to use a systematic method for examining key aspects of the study in order to make an informed judgment about the quality, validity and applicability of the study (see Ch 5 for a review of critical appraisal techniques).

One difficulty for guideline users when appraising guidelines for use in practice is inconsistency in the way in which guideline developers rate the quality of evidence and grade the strength of recommendations (Guyatt et al 2008). The need for transparency in this process is critical. After a review of existing models and frameworks used for grading the quality and strength of evidence systems highlighted inconsistencies and ambiguities leading to different conclusions, Atkins et al (2004) developed and piloted the Grades of Recommendation, Assessment, Development and Evaluation (GRADE) system. The GRADE system makes grading quality and strength two distinct components. Clinical guidelines are only as good as the evidence and judgments upon which they are based, and the GRADE approach aims at making it easier for users to assess the judgments behind recommendations (Guyatt et al 2008).

It is also important to be able to synthesise the evidence in the most appropriate way (e.g. meta-analysis or metasynthesis) to determine the effect of the interventions. Several methods and tools for critically appraising specific study designs and combining study results are freely available on the internet through organisations that provide education in EBP and develop evidence-based guidelines (see Table 4.3).

The process of formulating recommendations from the available evidence is not always straightforward, despite systems in place for grading quality. Study quality and results can potentially be interpreted in different ways by different members of the guideline development team. In addition, there may be insufficient research available, in which case the guideline development team must be forced to rely on recommendations based on expert consensus. The team must, therefore, have simple systems in place to obtain consensus of the recommendations and it must be made explicit whether the recommendations are evidence-based or consensus-based. Once the evidence to support recommendations is obtained, it can be incorporated into the guideline document. This document should outline the entire guideline development process from the need for the guideline to the way the guideline will be evaluated for effectiveness.

4.6.4 Apply and implement the guideline

Guidelines do not implement themselves (Field & Lohr 1992). Just because a clinical guideline is available does not guarantee its uptake in practice. In order for clinical guidelines to be effective, they must be perceived as useful and they must be used.

> [Clinicians] will criticise new guidelines for novelty, old ones for age, complicated guidelines for complexity, brief guidelines for simplicity, broad guidelines for lack of specificity, narrow ones for depth, visual guidelines for over-simplicity and written guidelines for verbosity (Dowswell et al 2001:122).

Strategies for dissemination and implementation of clinical guidelines depend on the local setting and the target audience (NHMRC 1999). A well-designed dissemination and implementation strategy is crucial to the successful uptake and use of guidelines in practice. Thus, acknowledgment of possible barriers to implementation, as well as strategies to overcome or minimise those barriers, is crucial to successful guideline implementation in practice. Although a recent systematic review of implementing clinical guidelines found no evidence to support a set or standard guideline strategy (Hakkennes & Dodd 2008), the reviewers supported earlier researchers in acknowledging the importance of first identifying specific barriers to change, and then developing tailored intervention strategies that deal with those barriers (Cheater et al 2005, Hakkennes & Dodd 2008). Examples of strategies that may be used for dissemination and implementation include:

- producing short summaries, printed and web-based
- incorporating the guidelines into local quality improvement processes
- presenting the guideline in user-friendly formats, such as algorithms
- piloting draft guidelines and incorporating feedback into the final document
- offering feedback on health outcomes and compliance rates

- targeting end users and involving end users in the development process
- using the media to publicise the completed guideline
- submitting press releases or articles to professional journals
- soliciting public endorsement of respected clinical leaders
- providing economic incentives, and
- using the educational processes of the organisation, local universities and professional organisations (NHMRC 1999, Robertson & Jochelson 2006).

4.6.5 Audit and evaluate the guideline in practice

Strategies for evaluation should be developed early in the guideline development process, as the success of a clinical guideline will be determined not only by the rigour of its development but by its actual use in practice.

Formulation of an evaluation and revision strategy will make the business of regular evaluation and updating of clinical guidelines less stressful. This information should be included in the report of the guideline so that the strategy can be followed consistently for subsequent revisions. Local peer review of the guideline document, as well as guideline use in practice, will enhance a sense of ownership and ultimate uptake of the guideline recommendations. The life span of a clinical guideline is dependent not only on prior evaluations, but also on new research and development. Therefore, regular revision is essential to ensure currency of the evidence-based recommendations.

4.7 Conclusion

This chapter has provided a process for guideline development and use. Clinical guidelines are available to assist clinicians in decision making, but should be used as an aid in conjunction with clinical expertise and judgment, as well as knowledge of the individual patient's values and preferences. To be of value, guideline recommendations should give clear-cut, practical advice about a specific health condition. They must be outcome-focused and evidence-based. Guidelines must be valid, reproducible, representative, flexible, adaptable, cost-effective, applicable, reliable and useful.

Clinical guidelines will always be susceptible to criticism and will never please all clinicians all the time (Dowswell et al 2001). Even a guideline developed using a rigorous and systematic method will not be suitable for all patients with the health condition of interest because of individual patient variables. It is important to remember the limitations of guidelines (Ricci et al 2006, Sniderman & Furberg 2009). Failing to reform the guideline process risks replacing one authority-based system with another, whereas the main objective should be to strengthen an evidence-based approach to improve clinical care. Therefore, evidence-based guidelines should not be considered the 'be all or end all', but should be viewed as a sound first step in the evidence-based management of healthcare.

4.8 DISCUSSION QUESTIONS

1. Describe six key qualities of effective guidelines.
2. What are nine guiding principles of guideline development?
3. Discuss a strategy for finding and appraising an existing clinical guideline.
4. What are the advantages and disadvantages of developing guidelines from scratch?
5. The guideline development process has been likened to the EBP process. Discuss the steps in the EBP process relative to guideline development.

4.9 **References**

Atkins D, Best D, Briss P A et al for the GRADE Working Group 2004 Systems for grading the quality of evidence and the strength of recommendations I: Critical appraisal of existing approaches. *BMC Health Services Research* 4(1):38–44.

AGREE Collaboration 2001 Appraisal of guidelines for research and evaluation (AGREE) instrument. Available: www.agreecollaboration.org 9 May 2009.

Browman G P 2001 Development and aftercare of clinical guidelines. The balance between rigor and pragmatism. *Journal of the American Medical Association* 286(12):1509–11.

Burgers J S, Grol R, Klazinga N S et al 2003 Towards evidence-based clinical practice: an international survey of 18 clinical guideline programs. *International Journal for Quality in Health Care* 15(1):31–45.

Cheater F, Baker R, Gillies C et al 2005 Tailored interventions to overcome identified barriers to change: effects on professional practice and health care outcomes. *Cochrane Database of Systematic Reviews,* 2005 Issue 3. Art. No: CD005470. DOI: 10.1002/14651858.CD005470.

Ciliska D, Cullum N, Marks S 2001 Evaluation of systematic reviews of treatment or prevention interventions. *Evidence-Based Nursing* 4(4):100–4.

Donabedian A 1992 The role of outcome in quality assessment and assurance. *Quality Review Bulletin* 18(11):356–60.

Dowswell G, Harrison S, Wright J 2001 Clinical guidelines: attitudes, information processes and culture in English primary care. *International Journal of Health Planning and Management* 16(2):107–24.

Field M J, Lohr K N (eds) 1992 *Guidelines for clinical practice. From development to use.* National Academy Press, Washington, DC.

Grant J, Cottrell R, Cluzeau F et al 2000 Evaluating 'payback' on biomedical research from papers cited in clinical guidelines: applied bibliometric study. *British Medical Journal* 320(7242):1107–11.

Grilli R, Magrini N, Penna A et al 2000 Practice guidelines developed by specialty societies: the need for a critical appraisal. *Lancet* 355(9198):103.

Grimshaw J M, Eccles M, Russell I 1995 Developing clinically valid practice guidelines. *Journal of Evaluation in Clinical Practice* 1(1):37–48.

Grimshaw J M, Russell I T 1993 Effect of clinical guidelines on medical practice: a systematic review of rigorous evaluation. *Lancet* 342(8883):1317–22.

Guyatt G H, Oxman A D, Vist G E et al for the GRADE Working Group 2008 GRADE: an emerging consensus on rating quality of evidence and strength of recommendations. *British Medical Journal* 336(7650):924–6.

Hakkennes S, Dodd K 2008 Guideline implementation in allied health professions: a systematic review of the literature. *Quality & Safety in Health Care* 17(4):296–300.

Harbour R, Miller J for the SIGN Grading Review Group 2001 A new system for grading recommendations in evidence based guidelines. *British Medical Journal* 323(7308):334–6.

Hayward R S A, Wilson M C, Tunis S R 1995a Users' guides to the medical literature. VIII. How to use clinical practice guidelines. A. Are the recommendations valid? *Journal of the American Medical Association* 274(7):570–4.

Hayward R S A, Wilson M C, Tunis S R et al 1995b Users' guides to the medical literature. VIII. How to use clinical practice guidelines. B. What are the recommendations and will they help you in caring for your patients? *Journal of the American Medical Association* 274(20):1630–2.

Keogh S J, Courtney M 2001 Developing and implementing clinical practice tools: the legal and ethical implications. *Australian Journal of Advanced Nursing* 19(2):14–9.

McSweeney M, Spies M, Cann C J 2001 Finding and evaluating clinical practice guidelines. *The Nurse Practitioner* 26(9):30–49.

National Health and Medical Research Council (NHMRC) 1999 *A guide to the development, implementation and evaluation of clinical practice guidelines.* Commonwealth of Australia, Canberra.

National Health and Medical Research Council (NHMRC) 2009 (last update September 2007) *NHMRC standards and procedures for externally developed guidelines.* Available: www.nhmrc. gov.au/publications/synopses/_files/nh56.pdf 18 May 2009.

Nightingale F 1860 *Notes on nursing. What it is, and what it is not.* Appleton and Company, New York, NY.

Osborne S 2009 Testing the effectiveness of a nursing practice development intervention on changing the culture of evidence-based practice in an acute care environment. PhD thesis. Queensland University of Technology, Queensland.

Oxman A D, Fretheim A, Schünemann H J et al 2006 Improving the use of research evidence in guideline development: introduction. *Health Research Policy and Systems* 4:12.

Pagliari C, Grimshaw J M 2002 Impact of group structure and process on multidisciplinary evidenced-based guideline development: an observational study. *Journal of Evaluation in Clinical Practice* 8(2):145–53.

Raine R, Sanderson C, Black N 2005 Developing clinical guidelines: a challenge to current methods. *British Medical Journal* 331(7517):631–3.

Ricci S, Celani M G, Righetti E 2006 Development of clinical guidelines: methodological and practical issues. *Neurological Science* 27(suppl 3):S228–30.

Robertson R, Jochelson K 2006 *Interventions that change clinician behaviour: mapping the literature.* Available: www.nice.org.uk/media/AF1/42/HowToGuideKingsFundLiterature Review.pdf 9 May 2009.

Schünemann H J, Fretheim A, Oxman A D for the WHO Advisory Committee on Health Research 2006 Improving the use of research evidence in guideline development: guidelines for guidelines. *Health Research Policy and Systems* 4:13.

Scottish Intercollegiate Guidelines Network (SIGN) 2001 *SIGN 50: A guideline developer's handbook.* Available: www.sign.ac.uk/guidelines/fulltext/50 9 May 2009.

Scottish Intercollegiate Guidelines Network (SIGN). Available: www.sign.ac.uk/index.html 9 May 2009.

Shekelle P G, Ortiz E, Rhodes S et al 2001 Validity of the Agency for Healthcare Research and Quality clinical practice guidelines: how quickly do guidelines become outdated? *Journal of the American Medical Association* 286(12):1461–7.

Sniderman A D, Furberg D C 2009 Why guideline-making requires reform. *Journal of the American Medical Association* 301(4):429–31.

Thomas L, Cullum N, McColl E et al 2003 Guidelines in professions allied to medicine. *The Cochrane Library* 1:1–43.

Webster J, Lloyd W C, Pritchard M A et al 1999 Development of evidence-based guidelines in midwifery and gynaecology nursing. *Midwifery* 15(1):2–5.

PART THREE

Locating the evidence

CHAPTER 5

Locating and appraising the evidence

David Gillham, Helen McCutcheon, Kate Deuter and Anna Holasek

5.1 Learning objectives

After reading this chapter, you should be able to:

1. plan a simple search strategy to answer a question arising from practice
2. identify and search databases relevant to nursing practice
3. locate relevant research articles using efficient and practical strategies, and
4. demonstrate beginning skills in the critical appraisal of research evidence.

5.2 Introduction

Nurses are required to provide care based upon the best available research evidence. However, all health professionals are confronted with an overwhelming quantity of accessible electronic information that must be evaluated for relevance and quality in the limited time available. This chapter will provide guidance on where and how to locate the best available research evidence, and describe efficient and effective strategies for the appraisal of the research located. To fully develop skills in this area, however, nurses should not only read this chapter but should also practice searching and appraising using the databases and appraisal tools described in this chapter.

5.2.1 Why is it important to develop skills in locating and evaluating evidence?

The quality of patient care is of primary concern for nurses and for this reason nurses must base their care and decision making on the best available research evidence. Basing nursing care upon misunderstood, outdated or poor quality research findings may potentially lead to adverse outcomes for large numbers of patients (Carr 2006). Decision making by nurses may be guided by a range of factors such as habit, tradition, instructions from other staff, intuition, experience, trial and error, prior knowledge and education, patient preference, policy and guidelines, and direct application of research evidence (Craig 2007). While research evidence may also inform education, patient preference, instructions from other staff, policy and guidelines, it is just one component of the knowledge the nurse brings to the point of clinical decision making (Kitson 2007, Estabrooks et al 2003).

It is important to remember that evidence-based practice (EBP) 'integrates clinical expertise and patient values with the best available research evidence' (Sackett et al 2000:1), and is 'a research-based, decision-making process utilised to guide the delivery of holistic patient care by nurses' (Boswell & Cannon 2007:10).

Given that nurses constantly have to make complex decisions, they are in fact applying research to practice continuously, perhaps without always being aware they are doing this. For example, drug administration is carried out according to the results of drug trials and is therefore research based. Similarly, there is a research basis for nursing practice in the range from complex wound care through to routine tasks such as pressure-area care. It is likely that busy nurses will correctly implement care that is based on research findings, but may not always be specifically aware of the research basis of their work. Thus, the use of research evidence is not a separate academic activity but a crucial component of hands-on practice.

It is equally important to recognise that almost all nurses and nursing students already conduct some form of filtering or appraisal of information. For example, when nurses hear or read information related to nursing practice it is highly likely they will automatically engage in an immediate assessment of the quality and relevance of the content. This may be as simple as assessing healthcare reported in a news bulletin or as complex as a careful appraisal of a research paper. Nurses reading research content may very quickly conclude that the information is valuable or, alternatively, not practical or relevant. Sometimes this evaluation may occur subconsciously and nurses may be surprised to be told they are already engaging in the evaluation of research.

Given the importance of appropriate application of research to practice, it is necessary to provide nurses with strategies to make sense of the overwhelming amount of information and research currently available. Nurses need simple and clear strategies for locating high-quality research evidence and, more importantly, they need to be skilled in understanding and critically appraising the information they have located. In addition to developing and improving skills in locating and evaluating research, it is important to consider the application of research evidence to practice.

One of the most critical tasks in EBP can be simply deciding where to start looking for the best available research evidence. Nursing students past and present will be familiar with the traditional paper-based printed resources—the nursing textbook, the professional journal or conference publication. While still important, and in some cases only available in print, these may not be the most useful resources for locating current research evidence due to the publication time lag (Dong et al 2006, Terio 2003). The huge growth in electronic publishing has meant the availability of the very latest, high-quality professional information and research, usually (but not always) available in full text and easily accessible via the internet. While finding information has never been so easy, finding the right information can be difficult and time consuming without some initial guidance. The information in Section 5.3 will help you to develop strategies for selecting the appropriate resources for locating the evidence you need, by introducing you to some of the key electronic nursing resources appropriate to your question or topic.

In summary, nurses must develop skills and strategies for locating and appropriately applying high-quality research evidence to practice. As discussed, a useful first step in this process is for nurses to recognise that they are already evaluating content and actively deciding to further develop their skills. The topics in this chapter present sequential and practical information aimed at helping nurses develop basic skills in accessing, appraising and understanding the best available research evidence. This will provide nurses with the best available evidence to bring to the decision-making process—evidence that can be incorporated with their own knowledge and experience in considering of the individuality of the patient. The challenge for the busy nurse is how to navigate the potential information overload and make sense of the information that is located. This chapter will discuss basic time-efficient strategies for the location and evaluation of research evidence while also offering direction and guidance for the development of advanced appraisal skills.

5.3 Where should I look for evidence?

It can be extremely time consuming to search the immense volume of published literature available in print and electronically, before locating and then obtaining the relevant evidence (Pravikoff et al 2005). Busy nurses and students need to become aware of the wide range of information resources available in order to make informed decisions about where to look for the best available evidence relevant to their question or topic.

When looking for current evidence, print-based textbooks may not be the best resource in which to locate the evidence because of the time involved in the publication process—generally 1 or 2 years. And although the internet is becoming an increasingly popular tool for quickly locating healthcare information (Gilmour 2007, Korp 2006), it is important to remember that there is no quality control of the internet and that:

> … the high-quality and clinically important sources are often hidden in a morass of information that is of questionable, or at least uncertain, quality (McKibbon & Marks 2008:34).

We need to be sure that the information located is credible, current and reliable, before determining if and how it can be used in practice. As nurses, we cannot afford to base our patient care on outdated or incorrect information. Fortunately, the internet also provides access to an increasing number of reputable, electronic healthcare databases and research organisations that provide current, quality, peer-reviewed nursing and medical research information.

> …because the steps of evidence-based nursing practice involve 'tracking down the best evidence' with which to answer a clinical question (Sackett et al 2000), understanding the resources available to nurses, as well as their skills in using them, is essential (Pravikoff et al 2005:49).

Thus, a useful starting point for this discussion is to introduce some of the major types of electronic sources of research evidence, such as databases and some specific search engines.

5.3.1 Databases

A database is a systematic collection of information that is stored, indexed, catalogued, updated regularly and able to be systematically searched. Databases can be categorised as either primary or secondary databases, although some databases may contain both primary and secondary content. However, in general, primary databases contain mostly original reports of research, such as those found in journal articles and conference proceedings, and are written by the researchers themselves (Pearson & Field 2005). CINAHL® (Cumulative Index to Nursing and the Allied Health Literature) is the most well-known example of a primary nursing and allied health database.

CINAHL and other important primary databases such as MEDLINE® (Medical Literature Analysis and Retrieval System Online) and EMBASE contain professional, scholarly, peer-reviewed journals, many of which can only be accessed after payment of subscriptions by university and hospital libraries. As well as providing access to nursing, biomedical and evidence-based databases, hospital and university libraries provide access to key healthcare print and electronic journals through their catalogues and through journal AtoZ title lists. It is important to note that it is common practice for publishers to place an embargo on accessing the latest electronic information (e.g. the last 6, 12 or 18 months). In these instances, the most recent information may only be available in print and not available electronically.

Secondary databases, on the other hand, contain summaries, reviews and appraisals of original primary information, such as systematic reviews, and can be found in the Joanna Briggs Institute (JBI) and the Cochrane Library, which is a collection of secondary databases. The location of systematic reviews is also addressed in Chapter 6.

Databases may contain links to full-text information, both full-text and citation information, or citation-only information, and may also include references to printed information.

Table 5.1 focuses on locating research evidence and, while not exhaustive, it includes a comprehensive range of online sources that can be used to search for high-quality evidence. How to appraise and apply this evidence is discussed later in this chapter. Because some of the resources listed in Table 5.1 require a subscription, and often a username and password, in order to access them, it is advisable to check with your university or hospital library as you may be able to access these databases through their institutional licences.

Secondary databases	What you will find
Cochrane Library	High-quality content • Cochrane systematic reviews • Other non-Cochrane reviews • Clinical trials • Technology assessments • Economic evaluations • Specialist Cochrane groups
TRIP	High-quality content • Access to a large collection of evidence-based material on the web • Articles from premier online journals such as *BMJ*, *JAMA* and *NEJM*
Joanna Briggs Institute (JBI)	High-quality content • Systematic reviews • *Best Practice* information sheets
PubMed Clinical Queries	Evidence-based answers to clinical questions • Produced by the US National Library of Medicine • Access to citations in MEDLINE, PreMEDLINE and other related databases • Links to online journals
BestBETs	Evidence-based answers to clinical questions • Evidence-based summaries
PEDro	Physiotherapy content • Citation details and abstracts of randomised controlled trials (RCTs) • Citation details and abstracts of systematic reviews • Abstracts of RCTs that have been critically appraised and rated

Table 5.1 Locating the evidence

Secondary databases	What you will find
OTseeker	Occupational therapy content • Abstracts of systematic reviews • Abstracts of RCTs that have been critically appraised and rated
NICE (UK National Institute for Health and Clinical Excellence)	Evidence-based guidance for nurses and other health professionals • Clinical guidelines • Technology appraisals
SUMSearch	Quality medical content • Searches the National Library of Medicine, Cochrane's DARE, and the National Guideline Clearinghouse
National Guideline Clearinghouse	Evidence-based clinical guidelines • Clinical practice guidelines • Guidelines databases need to be used with caution and assessed for relevance to the local context • Content is variable as minimal criteria for quality are applied to guidelines and it may be difficult to precisely determine the evidence basis for all listed guidelines
Primary databases	**What you will find**
CINAHL	Nursing content (as well as biomedicine and allied health disciplines) • Healthcare books, nursing dissertations, conference proceedings, standards of practice, educational software, audiovisuals and book chapters • Links to full-text journals, legal cases, clinical innovations, critical pathways, drug records, research instruments and clinical trials • Qualitative and quantitative information
MEDLINE	Biomedical content • Primary research papers • Links to full-text journal articles
EMBASE	Biomedical and pharmaceutical content, with selective nursing content • Primary research papers • Links to full-text journal articles
PsycINFO	Psychology content (and related disciplines) • Peer-reviewed citations, summaries and full-text links to scholarly journal articles, book chapters, books and dissertations • Qualitative and quantitative information
Science Citation Index (via Web of Knowledge)	Multidisciplinary (sciences) content • Searchable author abstracts
Current Contents Connect (via Web of Knowledge)	Multidisciplinary content • Tables of contents for journal articles, reviews, editorials, corrections, conference proceedings • Qualitative and quantitative information

Table 5.1 Locating the evidence—cont'd

5.3.2 Search engines

Popular search engines such as Google and Yahoo are software programs that only retrieve information found on the web and should be used with caution. Search engines vary considerably in terms of their coverage of the web, how frequently they update the websites visited, and the search options offered. In order to retrieve more relevant results, using the advanced search feature is recommended where available. Google Advanced Scholar search allows you to search for phrases, as well as synonyms or related terms, for authors and in named publications to retrieve fewer but more precise results. The instructions available on the advanced search or help pages are also useful.

It is not uncommon to locate an article of interest when using a search engine and then find that the full text is only available at a cost. When this happens, search for your article using the citation details in an appropriate primary or secondary database, or contact your hospital or university library.

While search engines can be useful as a quick reference tool, caution is needed in relation to the accuracy and credibility of the information obtained, particularly if healthcare is to be based upon the information found. Search engines will not necessarily retrieve peer-reviewed content (peer-reviewed content is discussed in Section 5.4) and while search engines such as Google Advanced Scholar retrieve better-quality information, there is much scope for further development in this area. Improved search engines designed to selectively access the highest-ranked evidence from multiple databases may be developed, thus allowing clinicians to locate evidence-based content easily. The TRIP (Turning Research Into Practice) Database can be searched in this manner.

Remember too that even though search engines may retrieve some full-text results, they will not find all of the information found in databases because they cannot be used to search systematically or comprehensively. In the near future, web technology and advanced search engines may improve not only the accessibility of research evidence for clinicians but also promote feedback from clinicians to researchers. However, at present, Google search results and Wikipedia cannot and should not be relied upon to retrieve credible evidence-based content.

5.3.3 Which source should I use?

Table 5.1 provides a list of potential sources of research evidence relevant to nursing practice. It is important to note that while these resources are well established, other resources may be developed in the future or there may be resources already of considerable relevance to particular fields of nursing that are not listed. Some workplaces and universities may also have licensed access to specific databases not listed here. Furthermore, while the resources listed are unlikely to disappear, their URLs may change over time. For these reasons, workplaces with internet access may find it useful to set up a small index of the most relevant databases. An excellent example of such an index for evidence-based health practice is provided by the Flinders University Library in South Australia (see www.lib.flinders.edu.au/resources/sub/medicine/ebm.html). See Chapter 1 for other comparable resources.

Constructing an index or portal of evidence-based resources is a useful first step in dealing with both information overload and content of questionable credibility. The next strategy is to consider which specific resources from Table 5.1 should be searched first. This will depend upon the reasons for your search and the type of question you are asking.

For example, if primary evidence is required, large electronic databases such as CINAHL, MEDLINE or EMBASE will provide access to the original study or the latest journal article. Secondary resources such as the Cochrane Library and the JBI provide critical summaries or systematic reviews of the best available research evidence (also discussed in Ch 6). A PhD student undertaking a research project would need to undertake a comprehensive search for evidence across a variety of resources, while the information required to answer a clinical question may be relatively quick and simple to locate using just one resource.

Having said this, it is worthwhile remembering that no one database is likely to identify all sources of potentially relevant data. Each database has unique characteristics, not just in terms of layout or display, but more importantly in terms of the content and the tools used to locate the most relevant information. To illustrate this point, let us consider and compare two useful, comprehensive primary databases for nursing: CINAHL and MEDLINE.

CINAHL provides indexing for over 2928 journals and contains 1.7 million records dating back to 1982. Examples of titles include *Journal of Advanced Nursing, Journal of Clinical Nursing* and *Journal of Nursing Education*. This database offers access to healthcare books, nursing dissertations, selected conference proceedings, standards of practice, educational software, audiovisuals and book chapters. Searchable cited references for more than 1200 journals are also included. Full-text material includes 72 journals plus legal cases, clinical innovations, critical pathways, drug records, research instruments and clinical trials. CINAHL can be searched by keywords or CINAHL subject headings; it also includes the Pre-CINAHL dataset, which provides searchers with current awareness of new journal articles.

MEDLINE contains bibliographic citations and author abstracts from more than 3900 biomedical journals published in the USA and in 70 other countries. The database contains more than 17 million citations dating back to 1965, including more than 130,000 population-related journal citations. Although the coverage of MEDLINE is worldwide, most records are derived from English-language sources or have English abstracts. Abstracts are included for more than 75% of the records.

MEDLINE is the electronic counterpart of Index Medicus®, the Index to Dental Literature, and the International Nursing Index. MEDLINE's controlled-vocabulary thesaurus contains Medical Subject Headings (MeSH®) to describe the subject of each journal article in the database and provide a consistent way of retrieving information that uses different terminology for the same concept. CINAHL is updated monthly, while MEDLINE is updated every week.

It is clear that searching multiple sources is always recommended due to variability in yield (results) for the search terminology selected and the unique collections in each database (Morrissey & DeBourgh 2001).

As mentioned, the question or topic being investigated will determine the type of evidence required and guide you as to where you can locate this evidence. To establish this, we can ask which type of research will yield data most relevant to the issue or topic: randomised controlled trials (RCTs)? qualitative data? systematic reviews? clinical guidelines?

Searching a large number of databases will provide comprehensive coverage. However, for practical reasons, it is advisable to restrict your searching. While the following three lists provide a starting point for searching, nurses may wish to add to these lists according to their specialty area or research interests. Common reasons for searching, as well as where to locate the information, include when you need to:

- *Quickly answer a clinical question*
  - PubMed: Clinical Queries
  - Cochrane
- *Investigate practice change*
  - Cochrane
  - JBI
  - CINAHL
  - MEDLINE
- *Research for academic purposes*
  - CINAHL
  - MEDLINE
  - Cochrane
  - JBI

- o TRIP
- o NICE
- o EMBASE
- o PsycINFO
- o SUMSearch
- o Science Citation Index (via Web of Knowledge)
- o Current Contents Connect (via Web of Knowledge).

Having searched for and located your information, the next step is to critically appraise the evidence to determine whether it is valid, reliable and applicable to practice. We will now explore ways in which to critically evaluate the quality of published content.

5.4 Is all peer-reviewed research evidence of high quality?

Assessing the quality of published research papers is not a simple task. Journals that publish research may be peer reviewed or alternatively not peer reviewed. Peer-reviewed journals are those in which the articles submitted for publication are evaluated by individuals who are expert in the subject area (Keenan & Johnston 2002). Peer-reviewed journals are often of high quality and are generally more highly regarded than those that are not peer reviewed. However, does the content of peer-reviewed journals always provide a suitable basis on which to change or ground nursing practice?

Peer review was traditionally regarded as a suitable means of quality control; however, this approach is no longer universally accepted as being adequate (Jefferson et al 2009, Frontera et al 2008). The most common peer-review processes used involve papers submitted for publication being sent to two or more experts in the relevant field to ascertain the suitability for publication. Problems may arise, for example, if the expert reviewers have strong clinical knowledge but are unable to detect problems with research design or the statistics presented. The result is that some peer-reviewed journal papers may not describe high-quality research design. This may not be the fault of the researcher, editor or author, but a consequence of limited research resources and difficulties associated with the complexity of healthcare.

A quick read of randomly selected Cochrane systematic reviews will invariably support this claim, as statements in Cochrane reviews frequently claim insufficient high-quality research studies on many topics. Unfortunately, this means that health professionals cannot be sure of the research findings from all published peer-reviewed journal papers.

5.4.1 Appraising the evidence

Nurses need to appraise research evidence before applying this to practice. However, developing skills in critical appraisal takes time and practice because of the need to understand both research design and how the research has been carried out within the individual study. There are many different types of research articles with different appraisal strategies used according to the type of article. This section discusses appraisal strategies and directs the reader to appraisal tools that can be accessed online and matched to the type of research article. It is important for students to practise using these appraisal tools (see Section 5.4.2.1) and share their research appraisals with work colleagues, students, educators and lecturers.

Fortunately, many internet content developers have recognised the need to provide access to simply presented, high-quality, rigorously reported research evidence designed specifically for use by busy health professionals such as nurses. This information is accessed via secondary databases, which contain content that has already undergone some form of appraisal. Remember, in contrast to secondary databases, primary databases contain content that includes original reporting of research studies, usually written by the researchers themselves (Pearson & Field 2005). There are many secondary healthcare databases, with a few of the more important databases discussed in this chapter.

Secondary databases that use rigorous appraisal processes, such as Cochrane and the JBI database, are extremely useful to busy health professionals because their content can potentially be used as the basis for practice, and the research evidence is presented as clearly and simply as possible. However, nurses still require appraisal skills to interpret this content. In addition, multidisciplinary review of the application of the research evidence to the local patient group will be important.

The Cochrane Library, for example, includes plain language summaries that convey valuable information clearly and quickly to health professionals and consumers. When reading this content, it is useful to keep in mind that often you are reading the rigorous synthesis of multiple research papers. However, despite the clear and concise format of plain language summaries, appraisal skills are still needed and careful application of research to practice is also required. Skills in using critically appraised evidence together with the development of skills in appraising primary research papers are essential and valuable approaches for nurses that complement each other. Critically appraised research such as Cochrane systematic reviews contain overviews or summaries of research evidence conducted over a set period of time; they address a specific question and are integrated by an expert team. Cochrane reviews provide the highest level of research evidence and as a consequence provide a highly reputable source of content on which to base practice. However, appraisal is needed even with Cochrane reviews. While Cochrane reviews use rigorous and standardised processes, the strength of the findings of a particular review is dependent upon the quality and extent of the research that was included in the review (Pearson & Field 2005). Furthermore, it is vital to consider whether the findings of the review apply to a specific client group and practice setting.

In addition to Cochrane, as indicated earlier in this chapter, there is a wide range of other databases that provide access to critically appraised content. However, some caution is needed when systematic reviews are accessed via journals rather than secondary databases. It is important to recognise that an article labelled as a literature review or review is unlikely to be a systematic review. Sometimes articles labelled as systematic reviews and published in journals may not meet the rigorous standards set by secondary databases such as Cochrane. Therefore, you need to look at both the title and source of the article and, even better, also conduct an appraisal using a systematic review appraisal tool. Table 5.2 provides an overview of commonly used databases that can support nursing practice, together with an overview of strategies for appraising research content located through electronic databases.

It should be noted that Table 5.2 provides a general description only and that the individual databases often contain a wider range of content than is illustrated in the simplified overview provided here. For example, Cochrane provides much more than just access to systematic reviews and the JBI much more than just *Best Practice* information sheets.

The right-hand column of the table discusses the need for a multidisciplinary and/or workplace review. There are several reasons why this is needed:

- An individual nurse may misinterpret research findings even from plain language summaries found in secondary databases such as Cochrane
- Any research findings need to be assessed to see if they apply to the local client group
- Change in practice may impact across multiple disciplines and therefore multidisciplinary review is necessary

Source	What you should do
Secondary databases	
Cochrane Library	• Read relevant conclusions and plain language summaries • Develop skills in interpreting content • If review findings are relevant to your nursing practice, take them to work as the basis for multidisciplinary discussion
TRIP	• Appraise according to the type of article located from within the resource • Conduct a workplace review
Joanna Briggs Institute (JBI)	• Read relevant *Best Practice* information sheets • Discuss workplace practice based on the evidence presented
PubMed Clinical Queries	• Appraise according to the type of article located from within the resource • Conduct a workplace review
BestBETs	• Appraise according to the type of article located from within the resource • Conduct a workplace review
PEDro, OTseeker	• Many studies are already rated using appraisal scales • Conduct a workplace review and assess the relevance to nursing practice
Primary databases	
CINAHL	• Use appraisal tools • Develop appraisal skills • Conduct a workplace review
MEDLINE	• Use appraisal tools • Develop appraisal skills • Conduct a workplace review

Table 5.2 Selective appraisal according to the source of evidence

- Appraisal is greatly strengthened if carried out by many health professionals, particularly if they have appraisal experience, and
- The use of activities such as journal club meetings may facilitate effective appraisal.

5.4.2 How can I use appraisal tools?

If five registered nurses are given a primary research paper to review it is likely they will identify diverse limitations and positive aspects of the given paper. While the process of gaining five different opinions and combining the expertise and experience of five nurses is valuable, using a standardised approach is likely to further assist the appraisal of research.

Critical appraisal tools provide a valuable approach to improving the evaluation of research evidence, although a recent systematic review of appraisal tools found limited consensus in relation to research appraisal tools (Katrak et al 2004). The appraisal tools discussed in this chapter are selected on the basis of clarity and relevance to specific research designs.

5.4.2.1 Where can I find appraisal tools?

Numerous appraisal tools can be accessed electronically. The UK Critical Appraisal Skills Program (CASP) (see www.phru.nhs.uk/Pages/PHD/resources.htm) has a range of appraisal tools for systematic reviews, qualitative studies, case-control studies, cohort studies, diagnostic studies, economic evaluation studies and RCTs (Ch 9 provides an example of application of the CASP RCT appraisal tool). Similarly, BestBETs has a range of appraisal tools that can be applied to varied research approaches. Given the range of appraisal tools available it is, of course, important to match the appropriate appraisal tool to the research design.

The PEDro scale developed by the physiotherapy department at the University of Sydney (see www.pedro.org.au), like the CASP RCT appraisal tool, helps to identify specific characteristics of research design that should be included in an RCT. The PEDro scale is particularly useful because the criterion for each item of the scale is explained concisely. In addition, the PEDro website contains appraisal scores for a large number of RCTs. A health professional repeatedly using the PEDro scale will soon become skilled in locating the content related to random allocation in an RCT report. Similarly, they will gradually develop the skills required to locate research evidence and answer the questions in the appraisal tool efficiently. An additional valuable tool for the advanced appraisal and reporting of RCTs is the CONSORT statement (see www.consort-statement.org).

The JBI provides a range of tools to assist with the appraisal of research evidence, with various licensing options available. These tools include RAPid (Research Appraisal Protocol internet database; see www.joannabriggs.edu.au/services/rapid.php), SUMARi (System for the Unified Management, Assessment and Review of Information; see www.joannabriggs.edu.au/pdf/sumari_user_guide.pdf) and QARi (Qualitative Assessment and Review Instrument). Further specialised JBI tools include MAStARi (meta-analysis), NOTARi (expert opinion) and ACTUARi (economic data).

5.4.3 What are the limitations of appraisal tools?

A useful exercise is to read a research paper, write down your initial impressions and then at a later time use a critical appraisal tool to evaluate the same paper. You can then compare your initial impression with your structured appraisal. This exercise is enhanced if it is carried out by several people or an entire class. The results of this exercise will depend on the paper selected.

Appraisal tools themselves are quite easy to criticise but difficult to write. An appraisal tool needs to have questions that relate to a multitude of different papers with a similar research approach. Therefore, many paper-specific aspects of appraisal needed for an individual paper may not be included. For example, a study may include an intervention and control, with the control consisting of routine care. It may be apparent to an experienced nurse that the intervention is far more time consuming and costly than routine care, and that this has not been reported in the study. Such a study could potentially score very well on appraisal tool scales even when the intervention is unworkable in terms of practical application. Situations such as the one described occur frequently and, as a consequence, it is important to remember that while appraisal tools are useful, intelligent independent review of the research evidence is also vitally important.

5.4.4 Overview: A simplified approach to appraisal

While appraisal skills take time to develop, nurses can improve their abilities in this area by using appraisal tools and attending or forming journal clubs. Acquiring such skills will be helpful in relation to understanding and applying research evidence. In addition, nurses can improve their use of research evidence by using content from secondary databases, particularly Cochrane and the JBI. While appraisal and careful consideration of the application of research evidence is still needed for secondary database content, this has in general already been reviewed. In contrast, primary content from databases such as CINAHL and MEDLINE generally requires thorough appraisal. CINAHL and MEDLINE, however, have the advantage of providing a comprehensive coverage of the published literature.

5.5 Examples of locating evidence

Section 5.3 outlined a number of useful databases in which to locate evidence to guide nursing practice. In Section 5.4 we discussed the importance of evaluating the quality of that evidence. Drawing on these two sections, we will now focus our attention on the practical realities of searching for and locating high-quality evidence. This will be followed by a detailed case study that employs the following search strategy. The strategy offered is not meant to imply a singularly best approach, but rather a snapshot of potential methods and tools.

5.5.1 Developing a search strategy

Before commencing your search, it is important to think about how you will go about searching for the evidence. Navigating databases can be a complex and often time-consuming task. Sorting through unnecessarily long lists of references can be minimised by starting out with a well-defined plan of attack.

5.5.1.1 Defining the question

The first step in undertaking any literature search is to start with a well-defined question. A research question should be framed in terms of the relationship between its clearly defined parts. For example, DiCenso et al (2005) suggest that questions requiring quantitative information (i.e. information about the effectiveness of an intervention or treatment) would typically consist of the following parts: the *population* (patient population); an *intervention* (such as a treatment, diagnostic test or treatment procedure); a *comparison intervention* (if any); and the *outcome* of the intervention. Questions requiring qualitative information would typically consist of two parts: the *population* (patient population) and the *situation* (condition, experiences or circumstances). This is also known as the PICO (Patient Intervention Comparison Outcome) approach, described by Sackett et al (1997) and Strauss et al (2005). The PICO approach was introduced in Chapter 2 and we will refer to it again at the end of this chapter in the case study.

5.5.1.2 Extracting keywords from the research question

Now that the question has a specific focus, examine it closely and extract some basic keywords from it (refer to the case study in Section 5.5.6 for examples). Single words can be searched as keywords in a database, where you are looking for the word(s) in the title, abstract or subject of an article. On the other hand, 'controlled vocabulary searching' (also known as 'subject searching') allows you to find all articles on a particular topic without having to search for every possible phrase or word that an author may have used to describe that topic. Controlled vocabulary searching will usually get you fewer results than the keyword searching option, but the results will be more relevant.

5.5.1.3 Limiting the search

Prior to commencing your search, it may be useful to seek the assistance of an experienced librarian. It is likely that a librarian will be well-versed in using a wide variety of limiters and can train you in their use. Furthermore, a librarian may also assist in highlighting and/or navigating the differences in spelling convention by checking the database thesaurus (a collection of all the index terms used by a database producer).

Once you are ready to enter some keywords into a database, you are also ready to decide which search fields you want to limit. You may want to limit the search to a specific time period and/or search for a specific type of article (e.g. research articles only). You may also want to focus on a specific aspect of your question; for example, causes, treatments or specific patient populations. Some common database search tools that can be used to broaden or narrow your search are as follows:

- *Controlled vocabularies:* Most databases can be searched using keywords although it is important to bear in mind that this method may easily miss other perhaps more relevant results. A more efficient and comprehensive way to search is to use a controlled vocabulary if available (such as a thesaurus or specific subject headings, as found in MEDLINE, Cochrane and CINAHL). Where a database includes controlled vocabulary or subject searching, it should be used if possible. If more thorough searching is required, then both types can be used.
- *Truncation:* Truncation allows you to search the root or stem form of a word with all its different endings. Using truncation essentially broadens your search. For example, using the term 'nurs*' will retrieve nurse, nurses and nursing (note that different databases and search engines use different symbols to truncate). A word of caution here—using this method can retrieve large numbers of entries that may be irrelevant to the specific topic. Note also that some databases and search engines now provide automatic truncation.
- *Wild cards:* A 'wild card' means that you insert a symbol (e.g. a question mark) in place of a letter in a word to pick up words that have different spellings, that is, US and Australian spelling. For example, inserting 'randomi?ed' would pick up both 'randomized' and 'randomised'. Not all databases have this function.
- *Boolean operators:* Another way to broaden or narrow your search is by using Boolean operators. This is done by inserting such terms as 'AND' and 'OR'. For example, a search for 'type 2 diabetes AND peripheral vascular disease' will only retrieve articles that contain both these terms. Similarly, by applying the operator 'OR', the database will find at least one of the terms.

In summary, if too many articles are retrieved, it may be necessary to narrow or limit your search. Likewise, if too few articles are retrieved, it may be necessary to widen the scope of your search, so that it is less precise. Remember, databases will become easier to navigate with patience and experience.

5.5.1.4 Retrieving the data

It is critical that you read the full-text version of articles. By not reading the full-text version you may miss significant details about the study population and how the data were collected (Munden 2007). Frequently, the full-text article is available at no cost. Remember that sometimes, however, the full-text article may need to be retrieved manually from the print form of the journal (see Section 5.3.1). If you are having difficulty accessing an article, it may be useful to seek the assistance of a librarian.

5.5.1.5 Documenting the search

Students often report wasting substantial time because they have not documented their own searching. Many databases allow the search history to be saved so that the search can be re-run without having to enter the same information again. It is useful to compile this information into a report form for future reference. Refer to the database 'Help' section for instructions on saving your search history.

CASE STUDY

You are a nursing student caring for Mr Allambee, a 50-year-old man with a 5-year history of poorly controlled type 2 diabetes mellitus. He is married with two children and is currently self-employed, owning and managing a small grocery store with his wife in the local town shopping centre. Upon his initial diagnosis, he was advised to lose weight and cease smoking, but no further action was taken. Despite numerous education attempts by the local general practitioner, his diabetes self-care management is still poor.

You now want to locate some evidence to support the provision of care to this person. How will you go about this? The first step is to develop your research question. Looking broadly across this case study, we can see that weight loss and smoking are two key issues for this patient. Previous self-management education has been unsuccessful. Let's focus on the patient's self-management education in this example and conduct a basic search. Using the PICO approach outlined in Section 5.5.1.1, you can begin to construct a very simple framework for the question:

- *Population* (patient population)
  - type 2 diabetes mellitus
  - male
  - middle age
- *Intervention*
  - education
- *Comparison intervention* (if relevant)
  - not relevant in this case
- *Outcome*
  - self-management.

More specific outcomes might also include:
  - weight loss
  - smoking cessation.

Using these terms, a broad question might be:

---

1. Defining the question

What is the impact of self-management education on males with type 2 diabetes?

Looking at this question, let's now extract some basic keywords. You can start by combining or connecting the following keywords with the Boolean operator AND:

---

2.   Extracting the keywords

- diabetes

AND

- education

AND

- self-management

Now let's enter your keywords into the CINAHL database. As discussed in Section 5.5.1.2, keyword searching involves looking for a particular word or phrase, which will usually pick up lots of results. In doing so, you retrieve over 500 results. Therefore, you need to think about the different terms and spelling that authors may have used to describe the topic (i.e. diabetes, type 2 diabetes, type 2 diabetes mellitus). So let's be more precise by inserting the following terms:

- type 2 diabetes
AND
- education
AND
- self-management

This retrieves over 150 hits—much better—but you still need to narrow the search focus to make it more specific. To do this, you can use the following CINAHL limiters:

3.   Limiting the search
Publication year: **(from 2005–2008)**
Peer reviewed ✓
Research article ✓
Gender: **Male**
Age groups: **Middle age 45–64 years**

By entering the keywords 'type 2 diabetes' and 'education' and 'self-management', as well as limiting the search to the above fields, you are able to narrow your retrieval rate down considerably. You find the following two articles particularly relevant to your search:
1. Nagelkerk J, Reick K, Meengs L 2006 Perceived barriers and effective strategies to diabetes self-management. *Journal of Advanced Nursing* 54(2):151–8.
2. Sprague M A, Armstrong Schultz J, Branen L J 2006 Understanding patient experiences with goal setting for diabetes self-management after diabetes education. *Family and Community Health* 29(4):245–55.
The final stages of your search are to:

4.   Retrieve the full-text version of the selected articles

Use the pdf icon if available to open the full text, otherwise you can use the *Linksource* icon if your institution has the software to link you to the full text available via another database. Depending on your institution, this may also be called by another name such as *Findit* or *LinkIt@Flinders,* for instance. Remember also to check your library catalogue to see if the journal title is available in print, and you may also be eligible to obtain the article through another library.

5.   Critically appraise the evidence

The next step is to critically appraise or evaluate the evidence to determine whether it is valid, reliable and indeed applicable to the problem or situation.

> ### 6. Summarise your search strategy

Let's now repeat this process, with the same question, this time using the Cochrane Library database of systematic reviews.

> ### 1. Research question
> What is the impact of self-management education on males with type 2 diabetes?

You can use the same key words and combine or connect your keywords with the Boolean operator AND.

This time let's also use Cochrane's 'Advanced Search' option.

> ### 2. Extracting the keywords
> - type 2 diabetes
> AND
> - education
> AND
> - self-management

To limit your search to look only for systematic reviews, use the option to 'Restrict Search by Product' and select 'Cochrane Database of Systematic Reviews' (Cochrane Reviews).

> ### 3. Limiting the search
> Cochrane Database of Systematic Reviews (Cochrane Reviews)

The Cochrane database is much smaller than CINAHL and your search therefore yields fewer but more relevant or targeted results. Note also that the more advanced search option of using MeSH is also available.

In particular, you locate two relevant, recent systematic reviews:

1. Duke S A S, Colagiuri S, Colagiuri R 2009 Individual patient education for people with type 2 diabetes mellitus. *Cochrane Database of Systematic Reviews, Issue 1.* Art. No.: CD005268. DOI: 10.1002/14651858.CD005268.pub2.
2. Hawthorne K, Robles Y, Cannings-John R et al 2008 Culturally appropriate health education for type 2 diabetes mellitus in ethnic minority groups. *Cochrane Database of Systematic Reviews, Issue 3.* Art. No.: CD006424. DOI: 10.1002/14651858. CD006424.pub2.

Once again, the final stages of your search are to:

> ### 4. Retrieve the full-text version of the selected articles

Systematic reviews in Cochrane can be retrieved simply by clicking on 'Record'. This provides access to an overview of the systematic review including a plain language summary, a more detailed version of the review and a reference list.

5. Critically appraise the evidence

6. Summarise your search strategy

As discussed in Section 5.4.1, Step 5 is to critically appraise or evaluate the evidence to determine whether it is valid, reliable and applicable to the problem or situation. Fortunately, Cochrane reviews make this task easier as the conclusions of the review highlight limitations of the research studies included in the review. In this case, both recent reviews highlight the need for well-designed RCTs. Also of interest is that the two studies located via CINAHL are not included in the reference lists of either of the Cochrane systematic reviews. This is most likely because these Cochrane reviews have quite specific and relatively narrow inclusion criteria. The Cochrane systematic reviews provide higher-level evidence relevant to our question than the studies obtained via CINAHL. However, the studies located via CINAHL also provide useful descriptive data. While detailed results from the primary studies retrieved via CINAHL and the systematic reviews from Cochrane have not been discussed here in detail, both databases provide useful information, and therefore in this situation it is useful to have searched both databases.

There are a multitude of situations that may arise when searching more than one database. The example provided shows the Cochrane database advocating further high-quality RCTs and a quick search of CINAHL retrieving useful descriptive data. More detailed searching of CINAHL is likely to locate studies included in the reference lists of studies included in the respective systematic reviews. In this situation, it should be remembered that the systematic reviews provide a higher level of research evidence. Conversely, it is important to remember that CINAHL may sometimes provide access to more recent primary studies related to questions for which there are not recent systematic reviews. Therefore, it is important to search both primary and secondary databases.

5.6 Conclusion

This chapter has provided strategies to assist with the time-efficient access of research evidence from electronic sources. It is not uncommon to find nurses who are prepared academically and experientially to manage complex patient care but not the complexity of in-depth clinical research techniques (Morrissey & DeBourgh 2001). It is therefore imperative that nursing students begin to develop these skills early in their academic training. Refining skills in searching the literature improves access to critical information, increasing the search yield and improving process productivity. Furthermore, effectively applying the skills of data review and critical appraisal to assess the validity of findings and improve patient care is essential to clinical practice development. While organisations such as Cochrane and the JBI facilitate the access of appraised research evidence, there is no better way to improve the use of research evidence than for nurses to further develop their own searching and appraisal skills. This improved understanding will facilitate safe application of research evidence provided there is adequate multidisciplinary review and careful consideration of individual client characteristics and the local practice setting (Livesley & Howarth 2007).

5.7 DISCUSSION QUESTIONS

1. What are the most important five databases for your nursing practice and studies, when assessed according to:
   - quality of content?
   - relevance to your practice setting?
   - level of evidence provided?
2. You are assigned the task of selecting electronic resources for a web portal in your nursing workplace (if you are a student consider a future workplace of interest). What will you include from the following list of possibilities, and why have you included these options?
   - secondary databases (Cochrane, TRIP, JBI, PEDro, OTseeker)
   - primary databases (CINAHL, MEDLINE)
   - other portals such as the Australian Centre for Evidence-Based Clinical Practice
   - appraisal tools (CASP, PEDro, JBI)
3. What is the best approach to appraisal of research evidence? You may wish to consider:
   - using appraisal tools
   - double-blind peer review used by journals
   - independent review by clinicians
   - using content that is already appraised
   - multidisciplinary review
   - seeking client input

5.8 References

Australian Centre for Evidence-Based Clinical Practice, Flinders University, South Australia. Available: www.lib.flinders.edu.au/resources/sub/medicine/ebm.html 19 May 2009.

Boswell C, Cannon S 2007 *Introduction to nursing research: incorporating evidence based practice.* Jones and Bartlett, Boston, MA.

Carr M 2006 Wound cleansing: sorely neglected? *Primary Intention* 14(4):150–61.

CONSORT Statement. Available: www.consort-statement.org 14 May 2009.

Craig J 2007 How to ask the right question. In: Craig JV, Smyth R (eds) *The evidence-based practice manual for nurses, 2nd edn.* Churchill Livingstone, New York, NY.

Critical Appraisal Skills Program (CASP). Available: www.phru.nhs.uk/Pages/PHD/resources.htm 19 May 2009.

DiCenso A, Guyatt G, Ciliska D 2005 *Evidence based nursing: a guide to clinical practice.* Elsevier Mosby, St Louis, MO.

Dong P, Loh M, Mondry A 2006 Publication lag in biomedical journals varies due to the periodical's publishing model. *Scientometrics* 69(2):271–86.

Estabrooks C, Floyd J, Scott-Findlay S et al 2003 Individual determinants of research utilization: a systematic review. *Journal of Advanced Nursing* 43(5):506–20.

Frontera W, Grimby G, Basford J et al 2008 Publishing in physical and rehabilitation medicine. *American Journal of Physical Medicine & Rehabilitation* 87(3):215–20.

Gilmour J 2007 Reducing disparities in the access and use of internet health information. *International Journal of Nursing Studies* 44(7):1270–8.

Jefferson T, Rudin M, Brodney Folse S et al 2009 Editorial peer review for improving the quality of reports of biomedical studies (Review). *The Cochrane Collaboration Issue* 1 1–41.

Katrak P, Bialocerkowski A, Massy-Westropp N et al 2004 A systematic review of the content of critical appraisal tools. *BMC Medical Research Methodology* 4:22.

Keenan S, Johnston C 2002 *Concise dictionary of library and information science, 2nd edn.* Bowker-Saur, London.

Kitson A 2007 What influences the use of research in clinical practice? *Nursing Research* 56(4):S1.

Korp P 2006 Health on the internet. *Health Education Research* 21(1):78–86.

Livesley J, Howarth M 2007 Integrating research evidence into clinical decisions. In: J V Craig, R Smyth (eds) *The evidence-based practice manual for nurses, 2nd edn.* Churchill Livingstone, New York, NY.

McKibbon K, Marks S 2008 Searching for the best evidence: part 1. In: N Cullum, D Ciliska, B Haynes (eds) *Evidence-based nursing: an introduction.* Blackwell Publishing, Oxford.

Morrissey L J, DeBourgh G A 2001 Finding evidence: refining literature searching skills for the advanced practice nurse. *AACN Clinical Issues* 12(4):560–77.

Munden J 2007 *Best practices: evidence-based nursing procedures.* Lippincott Williams & Wilkins, Philadelphia, PA.

Pearson A, Field J 2005 The systematic review process. In: M Courtney (ed) *Evidence for nursing practice.* Elsevier, Sydney.

PEDro. Available: www.pedro.org.au 14 May 2009.

Pravikoff D, Tanner A, Pierce S 2005 Readiness of US nurses for evidence-based practice. *American Journal of Nursing* 105(9):40–51.

RAPid. Available: www.joannabriggs.edu.au/services/rapid.php 14 May 2009.

Sackett D L, Richardson W S, Rosenberg W et al 1997 *Evidence-based medicine: how to practice and teach EBM.* Churchill Livingstone, New York, NY.

Sackett D, Strauss S, Richardson W et al 2000 *Evidence-based medicine: how to practice and teach EBM,* 2nd edn. Churchill Livingstone, Edinburgh.

Strauss S, Richardson W, Glazsiou P et al 2005 *Evidence-based medicine: how to practice and teach EBM, 3rd edn.* Elsevier Churchill Livingstone, Edinburgh.

SUMARi. Available: www.joannabriggs.edu.au/pdf/sumari_user_guide.pdf 14 May 2009.

Terio R 2003 Electronic metaphors and paper realities. *Progressive Librarian* 21:28–38.

CHAPTER 6

The systematic review process

Alan Pearson and John Field

6.1 Learning objectives

After reading this chapter, you should be able to:

1. explain what is meant by a systematic review
2. construct an answerable question on which a systematic review could be conducted
3. understand how to conduct a systematic review, and
4. discuss the importance and effects of taking account of both quantitative and qualitative evidence.

6.2 Introduction

The systematic review is critically important in the process of identifying the evidence on which to base practice. This is the tool that is used to locate the evidence and it involves the distillation from the literature of all of the evidence that exists for a given topic. In many respects, the systematic review is one of the great contributions to practice of the evidence-based practice (EBP) movement, because it recognises that with the burgeoning healthcare literature—some 2 million new items each year—no practitioner can afford the time to keep abreast of it all, even if they had the ability. Systematic reviews have relieved practitioners to some extent of this burden because they bring together and assess all available evidence.

Before launching into a detailed consideration of the process of conducting a systematic review, it may help to clearly locate this step in the overall process of EBP. The steps involved in EBP are:

1. identification of an intervention, activity or phenomenon
2. determining the best available international evidence on this intervention, activity or phenomenon through a *rigorous process of systematic review*
3. development of recommendations for practice based on this evidence
4. development of practice guidelines based on this evidence together with local consensus

5. implementation of these guidelines, and
6. evaluation of the impact of these guidelines on the outcomes achieved by use of the intervention in accordance with the guidelines.

The systematic review (step 2) is a fundamental step in the process of EBP. It is, however, a detailed process that involves a significant commitment of time and other resources. This is particularly true if the review is to be exhaustive, and there is little point to a review that is otherwise. Busy practitioners rarely manage to keep abreast of all of the current developments in their area of practice, much less have the opportunity to engage as individuals in the process of conducting a systematic review. Consequently, there are a large number of groups across the world that facilitate this process. There are a growing number of specialist collaborations, institutes and centres with skilled staff employed to train systematic reviewers, conduct systematic reviews and facilitate collaboration between reviewers.

6.3 **The systematic review process**

The systematic review is a form of research; indeed, it is frequently referred to as 'secondary research' (this is a reference to the source of data). Primary research involves the design and conduct of a study, including the collection of primary data from patients and clients, and its analysis and interpretation. The systematic review also collects and analyses data—but usually from published and unpublished reports of completed research. Thus, the systematic reviewer uses a secondary source of data.

As in any research endeavour, the beginning point in the systematic review is the development of a proposal or protocol. After a subject is identified, protocol development begins with an initial search of databases of systematic review protocols and reports to establish whether or not a recent review report exists: the Cochrane Library and the Joanna Briggs Institute (JBI) Library of Systematic Reviews are the most useful databases. If a review has been conducted, it will almost certainly be found in one of these two databases. If the topic has not been the subject of a systematic review, a review protocol is developed.

6.3.1 **Developing the review protocol**

As in any research endeavour, the development of a rigorous research proposal or protocol is vital for a high-quality systematic review. The review protocol provides a predetermined plan to ensure scientific rigour and minimise potential bias. It also allows for periodic updating of the review if necessary. The following description of the development of a review protocol may seem overly prescriptive, but these are the steps that are required to ensure a high-quality review. Given that the consumers of the review are likely to be relying on it for evidence upon which to base their practice, it is vital that the review is of the highest possible quality. The development of a high-quality protocol requires the following:

- *Background review:* The initial step is to undertake a quick, general evaluation of the literature to determine the scope and quantity of the primary research, to search for any existing reviews and to identify issues of importance.
- *Objectives:* As with any research, it is important to have a clear question. The protocol should state in detail the questions or hypotheses that will be pursued in the review. Questions should be specific regarding the patients, setting, interventions and outcomes to be investigated.
- *Inclusion criteria:* The protocol must describe the criteria that will be used to select the literature. The inclusion criteria should address the participants of the primary studies, the intervention or activity, and the outcomes. In addition to this, it

should also specify what research methodologies will be considered for inclusion in the review (e.g. randomised controlled trials [RCTs], clinical trials, case studies, interpretive studies).

- *Search strategy:* The protocol should provide a detailed strategy that will be used to identify all relevant literature within an agreed time frame. This should include databases and bibliographies that will be searched and the search terms that will be used.
- *Assessment criteria:* It is important to assess the quality of the research to minimise the risk of an inconclusive review resulting from excessive variation in the quality of the studies. The protocol must therefore describe how the validity of primary studies will be assessed and any exclusion criteria based on quality considerations.
- *Data extraction:* It is necessary to extract data from the primary research regarding the participants, the intervention, the outcome measures and the results. An effective way of systematically extracting data is to use a written protocol. An example of a protocol is shown in Figure 6.1. The protocol should be included as part of the report in order to afford transparency in method of extraction.
- *Data synthesis:* It is important to combine the literature in an appropriate manner when producing a report. Statistical analysis (meta-analysis) or textual analysis (metasynthesis) may or may not be used, and will depend on the nature and quality of studies included in the review. While it may not be possible to state exactly what analysis will be undertaken, the general approach should be included in the protocol.

The review protocol reproduced in Figure 6.1 is that used by the JBI.

6.3.2 Asking answerable questions

The assumption of EBP is that there are things we need to know in order to conduct our practice professionally. There are, however, substantial gaps in the knowledge available to us. Systematic reviews aim to expose the gaps in specific areas and provide pointers to the kinds of questions for which we need to find answers.

Sackett et al (1997:22) argue that almost every time a medical practitioner encounters a patient they will require new information about some aspect of their diagnosis, prognosis or management. This is no less true for other health professionals. They note that there will be times when the question will be self-evident or the information will be readily accessible. This is increasingly the case as sophisticated information technology gets nearer and nearer to the bedside. Even so, there will be many occasions when neither condition prevails and there will be a need to ask an answerable question and to locate the best available external evidence. This requires considerably more time and effort than most health professionals have at their disposal and the result is that most of our information needs go unmet.

The first step is to have a question that is answerable. Asking answerable questions is not as easy as it sounds, but it is a skill that can be learned. Sackett et al (1997:30) offer some useful advice in the context of evidence-based medicine and the effectiveness of interventions. These sources can be extended beyond questions of effectiveness, to consider the appropriateness and feasibility of practices. The source of a clinical question (adapted from Sackett et al 1997) includes:

- *Assessment*: how to properly gather and interpret findings from the history and physical examination and care
- *Aetiology*: how to identify causes for problems

Title:

Background:

Objectives:

Criteria for considering studies for this review:

Types of participants:

Types of intervention:

Types of outcome measures:

Types of studies:

Search strategy for identification of studies:

Methods of the review:

Selecting studies for inclusion:

Assessment of quality:

Methods used to collect data from included studies:

Methods used to synthesise data:

Date review to commence:

Date review to complete:

Figure 6.1 The Joanna Briggs Institute review protocol
Reproduced with the permission of the Joanna Briggs Institute

- *Differential diagnosis*: when considering the possible causes of a patient's clinical problems, how to rank them by likelihood, seriousness and treatability
- *Diagnostic tests*: how to select and interpret diagnostic tests to confirm or exclude a diagnosis, based on considering, for example, their precision, accuracy, acceptability, expense and safety
- *Prognosis*: how to gauge the patient's likely clinical course and anticipate likely problems associated with the particular disease and social context of the person

- *Therapy*: how to select therapies to offer patients that do more good than harm and that are worth the efforts and cost of using them
- *Prevention*: how to reduce the chance of ill health by identifying and modifying risk factors, and how to detect early problems by screening and patient education
- *Meaningfulness*: how to understand the experience of patients and the social context within which practice takes place
- *Feasibility*: how practical it is to implement a practice within a given clinical setting, culture or country, and
- *Self-improvement*: how to keep up to date, improve your clinical skills and run a better, more efficient clinical service.

Drawing on this, a clear, well-formulated question is developed to give focus to the systematic review. A clearly defined question should include specific details on:

- *Participants:* Participants should be defined clearly and this should include their condition (e.g. people with a confirmed diagnosis of emphysema), the population characteristics (e.g. females aged 15–20 years), and the setting (e.g. in hospital medical wards).
- *Activities or interventions:* The question should specify the intervention or activity of interest (e.g. chest percussion or the administration of oxygen via a facemask).
- *Outcomes that are of interest:* The question should include the outcomes of interest to the review. The patient's satisfaction with care, peak flow or oxygen saturation levels are examples of the kinds of outcomes one might include in a review of interventions aimed at improving outcomes in people with emphysema.
- *Types of studies relevant to answering the question:* The question itself usually indicates the study designs that will be most appropriate. When the question focuses on experiences of people or communities, interpretive studies are usually indicated, whereas questions of feasibility may warrant economic evaluations and/ or critical designs or evaluative designs. When the focus is on the effectiveness of a treatment, RCTs are considered to be the most appropriate, while questions relating to aetiology or risk factors may be best addressed by case-control and cohort studies.

Generally speaking, although health professionals often want to answer very broad questions, the narrower a question is, the easier it is to conduct the review. If the reviewers are interested in finding out the most effective, appropriate and feasible way of improving the quality of life for people with emphysema, it is desirable to conduct a series of reviews based on specific, focused questions rather than a broad, all-encompassing review that includes different populations, interventions and outcomes.

A well-formulated question will give direction to the search strategy to be pursued when undertaking a systematic review. See Chapter 5 for further discussion on asking a research question.

6.3.3 Finding the evidence

After you have identified the question, issue or problem from the field, the next step is finding the evidence. In order to do this, it is necessary to have knowledge about the techniques used to unearth the evidence and make it available. Although systematic reviews and practice guidelines are designed to save practitioners time by presenting condensed information, it is important that these summaries of information are open to assessment. This can only be achieved by accessing the process used in the review. Just as research—published or unpublished—varies in quality, so can a literature search. Practitioners who want to base their practice on the best available knowledge need to learn new skills to access the resources available to help them.

6.3.3.1 The logistics of a search

In developing your search strategy, and then implementing that strategy, the logistics need to be well thought through. It is useful to be clear about the following:

- What databases/resources can be searched? Not all databases are accessible to reviewers and only those that can reasonably be utilised should be included.
- Who will do the search? Doing a comprehensive search is time-consuming, laborious and requires a degree of commitment. Someone who has the time, skill and commitment needs to be identified to do this, and a second reviewer with similar characteristics is also required.
- What help will be available from librarians? Although librarians may not be well versed in the substantive area of the review question, they are highly skilled in electronic searching and in the retrieval of papers. Conducting a search without the help of a librarian is not recommended.

The search strategy should be clearly described in the review protocol. Determining rigorous procedures for the search before commencing the review reduces the risks of error and bias. The first step in any search strategy is defining preliminary search terms or keywords, and then using these to search appropriate electronic databases. The preliminary search enables the reviewers to identify other keywords and to modify them according to the thesaurus used in each database. Databases most frequently used are:

- *CINAHL®:* The Cumulative Index to Nursing and Allied Health (CINAHL) database provides authoritative coverage of the literature related to nursing and allied health. In total, more than 2928 journals are regularly indexed; online abstracts are available for more than 800 of these titles.
- *MEDLINE®:* MEDLINE is widely recognised as the best source for bibliographic and abstract coverage of the biomedical literature. It contains more than 17 million records from more than 3900 journals published in the USA and in 70 other countries. Abstracts are included for more than 75% of the records.
- *The Cochrane Library*
- *PsycINFO*
- *Current Contents Connect:* This is an index of journal articles, reviews, meeting abstracts and editorials. It covers more than 7500 international journals of all disciplines, bibliographic information including English-language author abstracts for approximately 85% of articles, and reviews in the science editions.
- *DARE*
- *AustRom:* This is a collection of Australian, New Zealand and Pacific region databases.
- *Science Citation Index*
- *EMBASE*
- *Dissertation Abstracts.*

See Chapter 5 for further discussion of some of these databases.

6.3.3.2 Conducting the search

As outlined in Section 5.5.1.3, searching electronic databases is complex and requires a great deal of skill. It is important to work closely with a librarian in deciding which databases to search and what search terms to use in each of these. A number of potential problems can be avoided if a skilled librarian is involved. For example, differences in spelling conventions such as 'randomised' versus 'randomized' and 'paediatric' versus 'pediatric' can be overcome by using the thesaurus of specific databases and using various other techniques. The same applies when different terms are used in different countries (e.g. 'mucositis' and 'stomatitis').

There are also variations in controlled vocabulary between databases. For example, MEDLINE uses the term 'cerebrovascular accident' whereas CINAHL uses 'cerebral vascular accident' to describe the same condition. Thus, when searching, it is important to utilise the aids available in databases. Truncation is an aid in some databases that can be used to search for a number of words with the same stem. In some databases, if an asterisk is inserted at the end of such a word (e.g. restrain*), then the search will include all words that contain that stem (e.g. restraint, restrained, restraining).

Another useful aid is that of the 'wild card'. A wild card can be inserted in the place of a letter to pick up words that have different spellings. In some databases, the wild card is used by inserting a question mark (e.g. randomi?ed) and any word with that spelling will be searched for (such as randomised and randomized). Most reputable databases have a thesaurus or controlled vocabulary, which is a list of headings used to standardise the indexing in the database. It is important to use this when conducting searches. It is also useful if you want to narrow or broaden your search to use Boolean operators. This aid is used by inserting the words 'AND' or 'NEAR' or 'NOT'. For example, if the term 'OR' is used between terms, articles containing either term will be identified. So, if you searched for 'mucositis OR stomatitis', you would get all the articles that had either mucositis or stomatitis in them. Searching for 'mucositis AND stomatitis' would locate only those articles that contained both terms.

Not all journals are referenced in the electronic databases and many other sources of evidence, such as conference papers and unpublished work, will be lost to the review if it is limited to only electronic searches. A comprehensive review therefore also includes manual searching of journals and the reference lists of articles and abstracts retrieved.

6.3.4 Appraising the evidence

After you have conducted an exhaustive search, the resulting titles (and abstracts, if available) are assessed to establish whether they meet the eligibility criteria set out in the protocol. Those articles that do not meet the inclusion criteria are rejected but bibliographical details may be recorded in a table for inclusion in the systematic review report. Some reviewers do not include this in the report (e.g. Cochrane Reviews do not do so), whereas others do (e.g. JBI reviews include them as an appendix). If there is uncertainty about the degree to which an article meets the inclusion criteria, or if the criteria are clearly met, then the full text of the article is retrieved. Two reviewers then independently review all of the retrieved articles. If both reviewers agree to accept or reject an article, the article is accordingly accepted or rejected. If there is disagreement between the reviewers on this issue, the reviewers should confer and reach agreement.

Although published work looks impressive and authoritative, it is important for reviewers not to view it as unimpeachable or sacrosanct. That is to say, all work should be open to scrutiny and questioning. No work is perfect, but some is positively shoddy, and shoddy work must be weeded out. To a certain extent, published work has been scrutinised if it is published in a peer-reviewed journal. However, it is most important that you are able to examine the work to identify what kind of evidence it has produced and how reliable or important that evidence is in terms of clinical practice.

Until 1999, evidence was ranked by quality in the National Health and Medical Research Council (NHMRC) *Guidelines for the development and implementation of clinical practice guidelines* in the following way:

- *I:* evidence obtained from a systematic review of all relevant RCTs
- *II:* evidence obtained from at least one properly designed RCT
- *III-1:* evidence obtained from well-designed controlled trials without randomisation

- *III-2:* evidence obtained from well-designed cohort or case-control analytic studies preferably from more than one centre or research group
- *III-3:* evidence obtained from multiple time-series with or without the intervention (dramatic results in uncontrolled experiments, such as the results of the introduction of penicillin treatment in the 1940s, could also be regarded as this type of evidence), and
- *IV:* opinions of respected authorities based on clinical experience, descriptive studies or reports of expert committees (NHMRC 1995).

However, as detailed in Table 2.1 (see Ch 2), this was modified in 1999 to read:

- *I:* evidence obtained from a systematic review of all relevant RCTs
- *II:* evidence obtained from at least one properly designed RCT
- *III-1:* evidence obtained from well-designed pseudo-RCTs (alternate allocation or some other method)
- *III-2:* evidence obtained from comparative studies with concurrent controls and allocation not randomised (cohort studies), case-control studies, or interrupted time series with a control group
- *III-3:* evidence obtained from comparative studies with historical control, two or more single-arm studies, or interrupted time series without a parallel control group, and
- *IV:* evidence obtained from case series (with either post-test or pre-test/post-test outcomes) (NHMRC 1999).

This hierarchy of evidence was designed to assess the validity of recommendations for clinical guidelines and focuses, understandably, on the effectiveness of treatment. Phillips et al (2001) have developed, however, a broader frame to assess levels of evidence related to therapy/prevention, aetiology/harm, prognosis, diagnosis and economic analysis (see Table 6.1).

This hierarchy of evidence takes a broader view of evidence but, like the NHMRC, renders all evidence that is not quantifiable as invalid for use in practice. Building on the Phillips et al (2001) framework, but taking a more inclusive view of evidence, Pearson (2002) reports on a hierarchy of evidence that includes the results of qualitative data (see Table 6.2).

6.4 The applicability of the evidence

There is little point in accumulating evidence to answer a question if we cannot then use that answer to benefit our patients. Remember, EBP involves the integration of best available evidence with your own clinical expertise. When it comes to deciding whether or not to incorporate into practice a particular activity or intervention, some or all of the following considerations will be relevant:

- Is it available?
- Is it affordable?
- Is it applicable in the setting?
- Would the patient/client be a willing participant in the implementation of the intervention?
- Were the patients in the study or studies that provided the evidence sufficiently similar to your own to justify the implementation of this particular intervention?
- What will be the potential benefits for the patient?
- What will be the potential harms for the patient?
- Does this intervention allow for the individual patient's values and preferences?

As well as needing to define levels of evidence for practice, there is also a need to establish levels of applicability. Pearson (2002) reports on the FAME (Feasibility, Appropriateness, Meaningfulness and Effectiveness) scale as a hierarchy of applicability of evidence (see Table 6.3).

6.5 **Software applications**

Most systematic reviews are carried out by specialist centres and overseen by experienced systematic reviewers with substantial research experience. The systematic review process is also usually managed using software applications designed for the purpose. Spreadsheet software such as Quattro Pro, Excel and Lotus, or database programs such as FoxPro or DataEase, are often used for electronic data collection and EndNote is increasingly used to manage bibliographical information. Review Manager (RevMan) and System for the Unified Management, Assessment and Review of Information (SUMARi) are programs designed to enable review teams to manage the systematic review process itself.

RevMan was developed by the Cochrane Collaboration. Users are able to enter a systematic review protocol, and then complete the review by entering information on each paper in the review (including the characteristics of each paper), developing comparison tables, and entering study data. Of most use is the facility to conduct meta-analysis of the data, whether continuous or dichotomous, from quantitative studies. This facility also includes the ability to present the results of meta-analysis graphically in a format that is internationally recognised. RevMan is downloadable, at no cost, from the Cochrane Collaboration website and is used extensively across the world (see www. cc-ims.net/revman).

SUMARi is a developing program of the JBI. It is designed to assist reviewers to conduct systematic reviews of evidence of FAME (Pearson 2002), and to conduct economic evaluations of activities and interventions. The package consists of five modules:

1. *Comprehensive Review Management System (CReMS)* is designed to accommodate the planning, monitoring and management of a systematic review. It includes the protocol, reviewer information, bibliographical information and time prompts. It incorporates the ability to import data from EndNote and includes fields to enter full-data extraction and full critical appraisal documentation. CReMS has the capacity to generate publishing-house-standard systematic review reports, and is suitable for researchers conducting systematic reviews that comply with the Cochrane Collaboration approach and for researchers who wish to incorporate other forms of evidence/data through the use of other SUMARi modules.
2. *Qualitative Assessment and Review Instrument (QARi)* is designed to facilitate critical appraisal, data extraction and synthesis of the findings of qualitative studies.
3. *Statistical Analysis Findings Assessment and Review Instrument (SAFARi)* is designed to conduct the meta-analysis of the results of comparable RCTs, cohort, time-series and descriptive studies using a number of statistical approaches.
4. *Narrative, Opinion and Text Assessment and Review Instrument (NOTARi)* is designed to facilitate critical appraisal, data extraction and synthesis of expert opinion texts and of reports.
5. *Analysis of Cost, Technology and Utilisation Assessment and Review Instrument (ACTUARi)* is designed to facilitate critical appraisal, data extraction and synthesis of economic data.

The CReMS module is web-based and, when downloaded on the user's server, can be accessed on the web by those authorised by the user. CReMS can be used as a stand-alone program or in conjunction with other SUMARi modules. Each of the other SUMARi modules are also web-based and are designed to interface with CReMS and all other modules.

The total package is designed so that each module interacts with the others and a reviewer can, at the point in the review when critical appraisal, data extraction and data synthesis/meta-analysis is reached, select a pathway to manage RCT data,

Level	Therapy/prevention, aetiology/harm	Prognosis	Diagnosis	Differential diagnosis/ symptom prevalence study	Economic and decision analyses
1a	SR (with homogeneity[1]) of RCTs	SR (with homogeneity[1]) of inception cohort studies; CDR[2] validated in different populations	SR (with homogeneity[1]) of level 1 diagnostic studies; CDR[2] with 1b studies from different clinical centres	SR (with homogeneity[1]) of prospective cohort studies	SR (with homogeneity[1]) of level 1 economic studies
1b	Individual RCT (with narrow confidence interval[3])	Individual inception cohort study with >80% follow up; CDR[2] validated in a single population	Validating[11] cohort study with good[9] reference standards; or CDR[2] tested within one clinical centre	Prospective cohort study with good follow up[13]	Analysis based on clinically sensible costs or alternatives; systematic review(s) of the evidence; and including multi-way sensitivity analyses
1c	All or none[4]	All or none case series	Absolute SpPins and SnNouts[7]	All or none case series	Absolute better-value or worse-value analyses[10]
2a	SR (with homogeneity[1]) of cohort studies	SR (with homogeneity[1]) of either retrospective cohort studies or untreated control groups in RCTs	SR (with homogeneity[1]) of level >2 diagnostic studies	SR (with homogeneity[1]) of 2b and better studies	SR (with homogeneity[1]) of level >2 economic studies
2b	Individual cohort study (including low-quality RCT, e.g. <80% follow up)	Retrospective cohort study or follow up of untreated control patients in an RCT; derivation of CDR[2] or validated on split-sample[6] only	Exploratory[11] cohort study with good[9] reference standards; CDR[2] after derivation, or validated only on split-sample[6] or databases	Retrospective cohort study, or poor follow up	Analysis based on clinically sensible costs or alternatives; limited review(s) of the evidence, or single studies; and including multi-way sensitivity analyses
2c	'Outcomes' research; Ecological studies	'Outcomes' research		Ecological studies	Audit or outcomes research
3a	SR (with homogeneity[1]) of case-control studies		SR (with homogeneity[1]) of 3b and better studies	SR (with homogeneity[1]) of 3b and better studies	SR (with homogeneity[1]) of 3b and better studies
3b	Individual case-control study		Non-consecutive study; or without consistently applied reference standards	Non-consecutive cohort study, or very limited population	Analysis based on limited alternatives or costs, poor quality estimates of data, but including sensitivity analyses incorporating clinically sensible variations
4	Case series (and poor quality cohort and case-control studies[5])	Case series (and poor quality prognostic cohort studies[12])	Case-control study, poor or non-independent reference standard	Case series or superseded reference standards	Analysis with no sensitivity analysis
5	Expert opinion without explicit critical appraisal, or based on physiology, bench research or 'first principles'		Expert opinion without explicit critical appraisal, or based on physiology, bench research or 'first principles'	Expert opinion without explicit critical appraisal, or based on physiology, bench research or 'first principles'	Expert opinion without explicit critical appraisal, or based on economic theory or 'first principles'

Grades of recommendations	
A	Consistent level 1 studies
B	Consistent level 2 or 3 studies *or* extrapolations from level 1 studies
C	Level 4 studies *or* extrapolations from level 2 or 3 studies
D	Level 5 evidence *or* troublingly inconsistent or inconclusive studies of any level

1 By homogeneity we mean a systematic review that is free of worrisome variations (heterogeneity) in the directions and degrees of results between individual studies. Not all systematic reviews with statistically significant heterogeneity need be worrisome, and not all worrisome heterogeneity need be statistically significant. As noted above, studies displaying worrisome heterogeneity should be tagged with a '–' at the end of their designated level.

2 Clinical decision rule (these are algorithms or scoring systems that lead to a prognostic estimation or a diagnostic category).

3 See note above for advice on how to understand, rate and use trials or other studies with wide confidence intervals.

4 Met when all patients died before the Rx became available, but some now survive on it; or when some patients died before the Rx became available, but none now die on it.

5 By poor quality cohort study we mean one that failed to clearly define comparison groups and/or failed to measure exposures and outcomes in the same (preferably blinded), objective way in both exposed and non-exposed individuals and/or failed to identify or appropriately control known confounders and/or failed to carry out a sufficiently long and complete follow up of patients. By poor quality case-control study we mean one that failed to clearly define comparison groups and/or failed to measure exposures and outcomes in the same (preferably blinded), objective way in both cases and controls and/or failed to identify or appropriately control known confounders.

6 Split-sample validation is achieved by collecting all the information in a single tranche, then artificially dividing this into 'derivation' and 'validation' samples.

7 An 'Absolute SpPin' is a diagnostic finding whose Specificity is so high that a Positive result rules in the diagnosis. An 'Absolute SnNout' is a diagnostic finding whose Sensitivity is so high that a Negative result rules out the diagnosis.

8 Good reference standards are independent of the test, and applied blindly or objectively to applied to all patients. Poor reference standards are haphazardly applied, but still independent of the test. Use of a non-independent reference standard (where the 'test' is included in the 'reference', or where the 'testing' affects the 'reference') implies a level 4 study.

9 Better-value treatments are clearly as good but cheaper, or better at the same or reduced cost. Worse-value treatments are as good and more expensive, or worse and equally or more expensive.

10 Validating studies test the quality of a specific diagnostic test, based on prior evidence. An exploratory study collects information and trawls the data (e.g. using a regression analysis) to find which factors are 'significant'.

11 By poor quality prognostic cohort study we mean one in which sampling was biased in favour of patients who already had the target outcome, or the measurement of outcomes was accomplished in <80% of study patients, or outcomes were determined in an unblinded, non-objective way, or there was no correction for confounding factors.

12 Good follow up in a differential diagnosis study is >80%, with adequate time for alternative diagnoses to emerge (e.g. 1–6 months acute, 1–5 years chronic)

Table 6.1 Levels of evidence and grades of recommendations (March 2009). SR: systematic review.

Source: Phillips et al 2001; updated by Howick 2009 (www.cebm.net/levels_of_evidence.asp#levels)

Level of evidence	Feasibility F(1–4)	Appropriateness A(1–4)	Meaningfulness M(1–4)	Effectiveness E(1–4)	Economic evidence EE(1–4)
1	SR of research with unequivocal synthesised findings	SR of research with unequivocal synthesised findings	SR of research with unequivocal synthesised findings	SR (with homogeneity) of experimental studies (e.g. randomised controlled trial (RCT) with concealed allocation) OR one or more large experimental studies with narrow confidence intervals	SR (with homogeneity) of evaluations of important alternative interventions comparing all clinically relevant outcomes against appropriate cost measurement, and including a clinically sensible sensitivity analysis
2	SR of research with credible synthesised findings	SR of research with credible synthesised findings	SR of research with credible synthesised findings	Quasi-experimental studies (without randomisation) OR one or more smaller RCTs with wider confidence intervals	Evaluation of important alternative interventions comparing all clinically relevant outcomes against appropriate cost measurement, and including a clinically sensible sensitivity analysis
3	3a SR of text/opinion with credible synthesised findings 3b One or more single research studies of high quality	3a SR of text/opinion with credible synthesised findings 3b One or more single research studies of high quality	3a SR of text/opinion with credible synthesised findings 3b One or more single research studies of high quality	3a Cohort studies (with control group) 3b Case-controlled studies 3c Observational studies without control groups	Evaluation of important alternative interventions comparing a limited number of outcomes against appropriate cost measurement, without a clinically sensible sensitivity analysis
4	Expert opinion	Expert opinion	Expert opinion	Expert opinion, or based on physiology bench research or consensus	Expert opinion, or based on economic theory

Table 6.2 Levels of evidence that include qualitative data results. SR: systematic review.
Source: The Joanna Briggs Institute. Available: www.joannabriggs.edu.au/pubs/approach.php#B 10 August 2009

Grade of recommendation	Feasibility, Appropriateness, Meaningfulness and Effectiveness
A	Strong support that merits application
B	Moderate support that warrants consideration of application
C	Not supported

Table 6.3 Levels of applicability of evidence
Source: The Joanna Briggs Institute. Available: www.joannabriggs.edu.au/pdf/about/levels_history.pdf 7 September 2009

non-RCT quantitative data, qualitative data, textual data from opinion papers or reports, or economic data.

SUMARi is marketed commercially by the JBI (see www.joannabriggs.edu.au/pdf/sumari_user_guide.pdf).

6.6 Conclusion

The systematic review process is one element of the many steps involved in an EBP model. A knowledge of the systematic review process is not only vital for those who endeavour to partake in the process of conducting a systematic review, but understanding the systematic review process is also of importance to healthcare professionals striving towards achieving EBP. This chapter has outlined the fundamental elements of the systematic review process and its importance to evidence-based information.

One of the strengths of a high-quality systematic review lies with the review question; a clear, well-defined research question will provide focus to the review. The steps to be undertaken in the review process should also be clearly described in the review protocol with particular reference given to the inclusion criteria and assessment of papers.

The appraisal of evidence is also an important aspect of the review process. Historically, papers have been given rank according to the NHMRC levels of evidence. However, as highlighted, not all evidence is concerned with effectiveness and many well-designed papers go amiss when solely using this criterion. The SUMARi package provides the necessary tools to assist in the appraisal and synthesis of all forms of evidence, from evidence of effectiveness to interpretive and critical papers, as well as papers founded in expert opinion.

Following the steps outlined in this chapter to conduct a systematic review will assist in achieving a high-quality review. It is important to remember when conducting a review that you are not alone. Enlist the help of others, such as a librarian, and the systematic review process should be a smooth one.

6.7 DISCUSSION QUESTIONS

1. Systematic reviews of research involve the meta-analysis of data derived from primary research. Is secondary research a legitimate basis on which to ground practice?
2. What are the implications of including qualitative research in systematic reviews?
3. Given that systematic reviews are being advocated as a mechanism for evaluating evidence for practice, how can clinicians assess the quality of a systematic review?

6.8 **References**

National Health and Medical Research Council (NHMRC) 1995 *A guide to the development, implementation and evaluation of clinical practice guidelines.* NHMRC, Commonwealth of Australia, Canberra.

National Health and Medical Research Council (NHMRC) 1999 *A guide to the development, implementation and evaluation of clinical practice guidelines, 2nd edn.* NHMRC, Commonwealth of Australia, Canberra.

Pearson A 2002 Nursing takes the lead: redefining what counts as evidence in Australian healthcare. *Reflections on Nursing Leadership* 28(4):18–21.

Phillips B, Ball C, Sackett D et al 2001; updated by Howick J 2009 Levels of evidence and grades of recommendations. Centre for Evidence Based Medicine, Oxford. Available: www.cebm.net/levels_of_evidence.asp#levels 15 May 2009.

RevMan. Available: www.cc-ims.net/revman 15 May 2009.

Sackett D L, Richardson W S, Rosenbery W et al 1997 *Evidence-based medicine: how to practice and teach EBM.* Churchill Livingstone, New York, NY.

SUMARi. Available: www.joannabriggs.edu.au/pdf/sumari_user_guide.pdf 14 May 2009

PART FOUR

How to evaluate clinical practice

CHAPTER 7

Undertaking a clinical audit

Sally Borbasi, Debra Jackson and Craig Lockwood

7.1 Learning objectives

After reading this chapter, you should be able to:

1. define what is meant by the term 'clinical audit'
2. understand how clinical audit fits within the framework of quality improvement
3. discuss the differences and similarities between audit and research
4. explain why clinical audits are useful, and
5. describe the major steps in the clinical audit process.

7.2 Introduction

Evidence-based healthcare has made huge inroads over recent years. There have been a number of bodies formed to produce and disseminate best evidence, and as a result a massive discourse has grown around the topic. Resources for quick access to information on best practice are plentiful and readily available to both practitioners and consumers. Yet, despite this mass of activity and expenditure in producing evidence, it has become clear that putting it into practice has been less successful. Indeed, uptake of evidence remains one of the key challenges facing nurses internationally (Borbasi et al 2008). The literature is full of interventions and ideas to help enhance the uptake of evidence into clinical practice. However, Thompson and Learmonth (2002:236) suggest that interventions such as didactic study days, and passively disseminated clinical guidelines and protocols, have 'little or no effect on practice'.

One tool that has been effective in advancing evidence-based practice (EBP) is the clinical audit. The clinical audit has been situated primarily in the final (fifth) phase of the evidence-based cycle and concerns evaluation. (The clinical audit follows after the first four phases of the evidence-based cycle, which are: formulating a clinical question; locating the evidence; critically appraising the evidence; and applying the evidence to bring about change.) Evaluation determines the effect of an intervention on clinical practice and patients. Thus, clinical audit is a tool to evaluate care and, with evaluation, the EBP cycle begins again (Mason 2002). Indeed, as noted by Mason (2002:295), any audit should be completed by follow-up audits.

This chapter introduces the concept of clinical audit as a tool that is increasingly being used in clinical environments under the aegis of EBP and quality improvement. The reader is provided with an overview of clinical audit as a way to develop knowledge and enhance clinical practice, including exploration of the usefulness of audit and of how to actually conduct one.

7.3 What is a clinical audit?

Clinical audit is a tool used by healthcare professionals to examine their practice and compare the outcomes either with quality standards, clinical guidelines or best practice evidence. In effect, clinical audit is a quality improvement process that aims to identify how to improve clinical practice, or to demonstrate that best practice standards are being met through current methods of care provision (Kinn 1995).

The primary goals of clinical audit are to improve patient care and related outcomes, and to promote the implementation of best practice evidence. The process used to conduct an audit can vary, but tends to be based on a series of related activities incorporating a number of steps—depending on the complexity of the topic chosen (commonly a four- or five-step process is described). Best practice or other standards are introduced to the practice setting, current practice is then audited and compared with best practice standards, outcomes are measured, and practice is changed if the audit results indicate a need for change. This process is repeated over time to ensure any changes to practice are maintained, and that patient outcomes continue to improve. As the ideal method of audit is to repeat it over time, audit has been described as a cyclical process that may be continuously, or intermittently, applied. A more formal definition of clinical audit suggests it is a:

> ... quality improvement process that seeks to improve patient care and outcomes through systematic review of care against explicit criteria and the implementation of change. Aspects of the structure, processes and outcomes of care are selected and systematically evaluated against explicit criteria. Where indicated, changes are implemented at an individual, team or service level and further monitoring is used to confirm improvement in healthcare delivery (NICE 2002).

Clinical audit then is a quality improvement and a change process based on the evaluation of current practice. Morrell and Harvey (1999:10) describe four main stages of clinical audit. The process begins by clearly defining best practice (stage 1); once this is established there is a move to implement best practice (stage 2), so bringing about change. This is followed by monitoring (stage 3) and comparing actual practice and outcomes against best practice standards (stage 4). Findings from this stage should lead to action to improve practice.

The National Institute for Health and Clinical Excellence (NICE; 2002:101–4) presents principles for best practice in clinical audit that incorporate an additional fifth stage. In addition to the steps described by Morrell and Harvey (1999), NICE (2002) include a stage for sustaining the improvements resulting from the practice change component of audit. The emphasis on sustainable change is valid and important given the varying effectiveness of ensuring worthwhile, long-term practice change in the care of patients (Walshe & Spurgeon 1997). The steps described by NICE involve preparing for audit, selecting criteria, measuring the level of performance, making improvements and sustaining improvement. These steps provide a framework rather than actual instructions for how to conduct an audit; hence, a detailed example is provided later in this chapter.

Shakib (2003) describes audit as a tool for determining the current state of a situation and, once results are determined, for bringing about change to best practice. Morrell and Harvey (1999) on the other hand refer to audit as a tool used to monitor and evaluate best practice after best practice has been implemented. Their model involves the development and implementation of best practice standards into care that is then followed up by audit. Either way, it can be seen that audit is really all about improving patient care. It is never static; both of the models described above include a need for continual re-audit. Audit is also a useful tool to establish a baseline for later comparison when considering change in practice. Baseline audits assist in identifying and prioritising areas of guideline-related practice that require change (Perry 2007).

After change has been implemented, repeat audits serve to evaluate whether there have been any gains from it. Perry (2007) points out that audit may be a way of convincing staff of the need for change, as it offers promise of evaluation, which is something clinicians often complain is not forthcoming. However, Thompson and Learmonth (2002:230) warn that on its own, clinical audit is probably not a sufficient mechanism for bringing about sustained change and that a number of multifaceted strategies for change should be put in place. These may include electronic or paper-based reminders and educational programs (Thompson & Learmonth 2002:236).

Though many clinical audits are conducted locally, Mason (2002) advocates national audits over and above local audit projects, which he claims, for a variety of reasons, tend not to produce better health outcomes. He states, 'the future of clinical audit, as a major agent of change, lies with nationally organised projects associated with national priorities' (Mason 2002:296). UK national audits have included the Myocardial Infarction National Audit Project and the National Sentinel Audit for Stroke, both of which have used the latest in information technology, rapid feedback to stakeholders and re-audit. Other national clinical audits undertaken in the UK include the management of elderly people who have had falls, the management of violence in mental-health settings, the management of patients with venous leg ulcers and audit of the use of caesarean section (NICE 2002:94).

7.4 How does a clinical audit relate to the quality improvement movement?

In an effort to improve the quality of clinical practice over the past few years, a number of initiatives have emerged, the names of which have changed as 'new groups of management gurus' have refashioned and reshaped former ideas (Mason 2002:294). Thus, terminology surrounding the notion of providing best care is dynamic. For example, until recently, clinical effectiveness has been popular, but now the wider concept of clinical governance has come into vogue. In the UK, Morrell and Harvey (1999:10) see clinical audit as part of clinical effectiveness and quality improvement, whereas Mason (2002) states that clinical audit has become an integral component of the clinical governance processes within the National Health Service (NHS). Both are correct. Clinical governance is the framework through which clinical effectiveness takes place, and is intended as an accountability model focused on creating environments that seek to safeguard high standards of care and continuously improve them (Gaston 2003).

Clinical effectiveness has been defined as:

> … applying the best available knowledge, derived from research, clinical expertise and patient preferences, to achieve optimum processes and outcomes of care for patients (Royal College of Nursing 1996, cited in Morrell & Harvey 1999:11).

Clinical audit is regarded as an integral part of any clinical effectiveness program (Morrell & Harvey 1999:156), whereas clinical governance is seen as:

> … a system through which… organisations are accountable for continuously improving the quality of their services and safeguarding high standards of care by creating an environment in which excellence in clinical care will flourish (Scally & Donaldson 1998:61).

It divides quality into four aspects:
1. professional performance (technical quality)
2. resource use (efficiency)
3. risk management (the risk of injury or illness associated with the service provided), and
4. patients' satisfaction with the service provided (WHO 1983, cited in Scally & Donaldson 1998:61).

NICE in the UK believe 'clinical audit is at the heart of clinical governance' (NICE 2002:vi). NICE have produced a book called *Principles for best practice in clinical audit*, which can be downloaded free from the NICE website (see www.nice. org.uk).

As described in Chapter 1, the National Institute of Clinical Studies (NICS) was established by the Australian Federal Government in 2000, and commenced operations in 2001. The primary purpose of the NICS is to champion continuous improvement in the quality and delivery of clinical practice to the Australian community. The methods by which this is to be achieved are based on partnership with consumers, health professionals, health organisations, researchers and governments. In collaboration with these groups, the NICS seeks to close the gaps between evidence and clinical practice in those areas that will effect significant change for the Australian community. It seeks to do this by providing practitioners and health organisations with systems that will assist them to improve the health outcomes of those within their care.

The methods used in the NICS projects vary according to the topic in question, although the focus across all projects is the implementation of evidence in practice. Evaluations of projects and programs initiated by the NICS reflect similarity to audit programs in that there are distinct barriers and facilitators to change. The challenge to address these in context-specific ways has been taken on by the NICS through the development of reference groups with the role of establishing a coordinated national approach to implementation. The parallels with optimal audit program design include use of multidisciplinary approaches, use of broad-based programs to target key clinical problems identified via research, and then use of multiple methods to close the gaps between evidence and practice. Details of some of the work of the NICS were presented in Appendix 1.1 in Chapter 1.

7.5 What do clinical audits measure?

The UK-based NICE describes clinical audit as a strategy to monitor the use of particular interventions or care received by patients against agreed standards (NICE 2002). Effectiveness is the degree to which an intervention does what it is meant to do in normal circumstances (Thomas 1999). In assessing effectiveness, evidence is needed to determine if intended outcomes were achieved. The clinical audit process is a way of ascertaining the achievement or failure of intended outcomes. It allows the identification of departure from best practices so they can be examined in an effort to understand and act upon the causes (NICE 2002).

Thomas (1999:41) differentiates clinical audit from medical audit by defining the former as being concerned with the 'total package of care offered to patients', rather than focusing only on medical care. The clinical audit focuses on nursing care, service provision and management, as well as physical and environmental issues (Thomas 1999). This positions the clinical audit as an essentially multidisciplinary activity, which is in keeping with the fact that the provision of health services is also a multidisciplinary activity (Closs & Cheater 1996).

7.6 Audit or research?

Nurses have been evaluating their work for years but have not actually called that process audit (Kinn 1995). In nursing circles, what began as medical audits have now become clinical audits (Mason 2002), and clinical audits have come to be viewed as an important aspect of professional accountability (NICE 2002:8). There is some contention over whether or not clinical audits are research and therefore require approval from an institutional ethics committee (IEC). Scott (2000) is convinced clinical audit is research, whereas CRAG (Clinical Resource and Audit Group) in Scotland categorically takes the view that because research is about establishing new knowledge, audit is not research (cited Morrell & Harvey 1999:3).

Balogh (1996) also points out that research is concerned with extending knowledge, whereas audits are concerned with making sure that best current knowledge is being applied in practice and promoting positive practice change. However, Balogh (1996) acknowledges the similarities between audit and research, in that they both engage in a process of inquiry, and both employ similar strategies for gathering and analysing information (similarly Mead & Moseley 1996). Closs and Cheater (1996) highlight further differences in the two processes, in that audit is theorised as a repeating, circular process, whereas with some exceptions, research is more often conceptualised as linear in nature. Furthermore, whereas much research aims to be generalisable, audits are carried out in local environments and therefore reflect practices in a particular setting (Balogh 1996). The nature of the clinical audit can be likened to the action research cycle, which also focuses on local solutions to local problems and engages in a process of data collection to facilitate practice change. The University Hospitals Bristol NHS Foundation Trust, through their Clinical Audit Central Office, has produced a series of short papers on different aspects of clinical audit, including one called *How to apply ethics to clinical audit* (see www.uhbristol.nhs.uk/healthcare-professionals/clinical-audit/how-to-guides.html).

No matter where one sits in the debate, it is clear that undertaking a clinical audit can contribute to research by drawing attention to areas requiring further research, as well as raising new researchable areas (Balogh 1996). Audit is a mechanism by which the gap between research and practice can be closed by comparing the two, identifying any inconsistencies, and guiding the development of methods to improve practice in the light of research findings. Despite the controversy, it is clear that clinical audits do raise ethical issues (e.g. use of patient records to gather information). Therefore, clinical audits should adhere to the same ethical principles common to any sphere of clinical practice, investigation or research, and require approval from an institutional body specifically set up to assess such proposals, such as an IEC (Morrell & Harvey 1999:105, NICE 2002).

7.7 Why are clinical audits useful in practice development?

There are a number of advantages to clinical audit. Ideally the audit should be a routine part of care (Closs & Cheater 1996) and so produce a constant spiral of intervention–monitoring–review of clinical care. Kinn (1995:36) notes that raising standards of care can only benefit patient outcomes and that the provision of care will be more efficient, which should enhance the job satisfaction of staff. Audit is seen to be educational and a useful tool for fostering interdisciplinary teamwork and communication. Morrell and Harvey (1999:158) state that clinical audit provides an avenue for reflection on work by healthcare workers, which, in turn, facilitates the development of their practice, knowledge and attitudes. The development of practice and the development of practitioners are regarded as inextricably linked (Morrell et al 1995, cited in Morrell & Harvey 1999:158).

NICE (2002) point out that effective clinical audit is important for a range of stakeholders, including health professionals, health service managers, patients and the public. They explain that audits:

- support health professionals in ensuring their patients receive the best possible care
- inform health service managers of the need for organisational change, or new investment to support health professionals in their practice
- assist in ensuring that patients are given the best possible care, and
- provide the public with confidence in the quality of the service as a whole (see www.nice.org.uk/media/796/23/BestPracticeClinicalAudit.pdf).

7.8 The process of undertaking a clinical audit

Considerations in setting up an audit include whether it will use a top-down or bottom-up approach, the time available, the need for extra resources and whether the audit problem is in an area where any changes will have 'a real effect on the immediate working environment' (Kinn 1995:36).

Morrell and Harvey (1999) restate that the fundamental principles underpinning a clinical audit are that it should:

- be professionally led
- be seen as an educational process
- form a part of routine clinical practice
- be based on the setting of standards
- generate results that can be used to improve outcome of quality care
- involve management in both the process and outcome of audit
- be confidential at the individual patient/clinician level, and
- be informed by the views of patients/clients (Department of Health UK 1993, cited in Morrell & Harvey 1999:2–3).

In conducting a clinical audit, there are a number of factors to consider. Shakib (2003:17) calls these 'audit fundamentals', and while some may not be compulsory they are important because they promote a carefully thought-out and systematic approach to the task. Prudent planning in the early stages makes for increased efficiency throughout the process.

Any clinical audit needs a written (or computer-generated) proposal. This information is used to apply for either ethical approval or perhaps to an audit committee, if that is the institution's policy. The proposal should include a title and a location for the audit; for example, 'Prospective audit of intravenous cannulations in Wards 5Y and 5Z'. The names of all the people who will be significantly involved in conducting the audit are included. These staff are usually those who have constructed the aims and objectives behind the audit and who have a good understanding of the issues involved (Shakib 2003). It is essential that the audit have 'a clear purpose and clear aims' (Shakib 2003:19), and so justification for its conduct is unmistakable. The specific outcomes of the project and the endpoints to be measured need to be spelt out, and consideration given to any factors that might influence the outcomes of interest. For example, it would be important to know how long cannulas were routinely left in place in Ward 5Y as opposed to Ward 5Z, and who was responsible for replacing the cannulas in each ward.

Inclusion criteria are the factors defining the population you want to study. These need to be carefully identified (Shakib 2003:21). For example, you may want to include only those patients who have cannulas inserted on the ward—not those who received one in the emergency department or who have been transferred from another ward/hospital. Exclusion criteria are those factors you are not interested in exploring (e.g. you may only wish to look at peripheral cannulas, not central lines).

Shakib (2003:21) suggests there needs to be some thought given to what the team thinks the audit will find. In this way, the outcomes and the factors that impact on the outcomes can be selected 'in such a way as to highlight the aspects of the results that you are interested in' (Shakib 2003:21). Shakib strongly reinforces the view of there being absolutely no point in conducting an audit unless there is firm commitment to acting on the results. Some pre-empting of what the audit may show allows the team to start thinking about intervention strategies and re-auditing. This means the team may opt to collect slightly different data in order to make the intervention/s and re-auditing easier (Shakib 2003:21).

The next section of the proposal contains reference to the methods you are going to use to collect your data. Shakib (2003) urges rigour in data collection. Morrell and Harvey (1999:49) refer to the importance of good measurement. Because there is a real probability the audit will demonstrate a need to change practice, the results must be believable, and data-collection and analysis processes open to scrutiny. When 'unsavoury' audit data are presented, staff tend to mount their defences and any weaknesses in the audit process are quickly spotted (Morrell & Harvey 1999:22), rendering results (and thus the need to change practice) much less convincing. It is important to remember that an overemphasis on rigour 'risks alienating the very people likely to benefit from involvement in clinical audit' (Morrell & Harvey 1999:49), and so the relational aspects to audit need to be borne in mind. Morrell and Harvey (1999:9) are quick to stress a collaborative, multiprofessional approach to audit and the benefits of the process to team building.

The sources of audit data can include, for example, questionnaires, interviews and direct observation, as well as pre-existing sources such as medical records, patient notes and discharge data.

Several aspects of the sampling procedure need to be determined, not least of which are how many patients are required and whether they will be randomly selected and in within what time frame. Other considerations include:
- Who will collect the data?
- Will it be retrospectively or prospectively collected?
- Will consent be required?
- How will the data be recorded?
- How will it be analysed?
- What unanticipated hiccups might there be along the way (e.g. non-compliant staff)? (For greater depth see, for example, Shakib 2003, NICE 2002, Morrell & Harvey 1999.)

After the data are collected they need to be analysed and a summary of the findings written up and presented to the clinical audit group for interpretation. The audit summary needs to provide constructive feedback, bearing in mind areas of both high and low achievement (Morrell & Harvey 1999:69). This is so that the group can look at ways to extrapolate success into areas requiring improvement. In this way, clinical audit becomes less threatening to staff and does not just focus on negative aspects (Morrell & Harvey 1999:70).

The next step in the audit cycle is often the most problematic and involves planning for improvement or bringing about change. This is where knowledge of change theory becomes important. There are many texts devoted entirely to strategies and theories to bring about change; they make essential reading for clinicians wanting to implement best practice. More recently, Cochrane has produced several reviews on strategies to effect change in the behaviour of health professionals. After change has been implemented, there needs to be regular re-audit and review (usually in 6-monthly or annual cycles). A report is often required and presentation of the project to a steering group or other interested parties. Publication to disseminate certain information regarding your audit is also a possibility. It is a good idea for the audit team to come together for some reflection on how the audit went and what might be done differently the next time (Morrell & Harvey 1999:84).

Organisational support for clinical auditing is paramount to its success and is increasingly being provided through the establishment of clinical governance suites in many Australian healthcare facilities. The most commonly cited barrier to successful audit is the failure of an organisation to provide staff with the necessary protected time to carry out the work (NICE 2002:153). In addition, institutions need to recognise that audits require adequate funding and that changes to practice resulting from audits can actually increase costs, especially in the first instance (NICE 2002:154). Yet, sustaining the improvements made to patient care through audit is essential to the success of clinical governance. Monitoring and evaluating change is advocated through re-audit and review. Maintaining and reinforcing change over time includes the need for:

- reinforcing or motivating factors to be built in by management to support the continual cycle of quality improvement
- integration of audit into the organisation's wider quality improvement systems, and
- strong leadership (NICE 2002:62).

7.9 **Example of a clinical audit**

In the following sections, the process of conducting a clinical audit is described drawing, by way of example, from an audit that has actually been completed (see Table 7.1). The framework used is detailed and can be used or adapted as required. This outline can also be used to form the basis of an audit protocol, which is a highly recommended component of the audit process. The benefits of writing an audit protocol are that it clarifies exactly the methods and structure of the audit, and enhances communication and collaboration with key stakeholders.

The remainder of this section will be structured under the following framework:

- Topic selection
- Question development and objectives
- Identifying best practice
- Audit indicator development
- Method
- Sampling and data collection
- Data analysis and evaluation
- Feedback
- Implementation of best practice (standard/s), and
- Re-auditing.

7.9.1 **Topic selection**

When selecting an audit topic, priority should be given to selection of topics in areas where significant improvements to clinical care can be made—achieving the best outcome for your efforts should be kept in mind. There should be practical ways to

FACILITY/WARD	CLINICAL AUDITING PROGRAM

AUDIT TOPIC:	Date:

Split-thickness skin graft donor sites: post-harvest management

Related Standards: JBI 2002 *Best Practice* information sheet 6(2)

Audit objectives: To measure the care interventions patients receive in relation to the post-harvest management of split-thickness skin graft donor sites.

Rationale: Clinical experience suggests that care is varied, and that patients are experiencing ongoing problems with wound leakage and multiple dressing changes.

Audit team: Clinicians and data collectors directly involved in the audit process.

CLINICAL GUIDELINE	AUDIT INDICATOR
1. The primary dressing is a moist wound-healing product. **2.** The size and type of primary dressing applied is appropriate for the anticipated volume of exudate. **3.** The primary dressing is left intact and reinforced if required for the first 24–48 hours postoperatively.	1. ___100___ % of dressing products applied will be moist wound-healing products. 2. ___100___ % of dressing selections will be based on anticipated volumes of exudate. 3. ___100___ % of primary dressings and reinforcement will be left intact for 24–48 hours postoperatively.

Reference: JBI 2002 Best Practice *information sheet* 6(2).

AUDIT INDICATORS

1. 100 % of dressing products applied will be moist wound-healing products.

Structure	Process	Outcome
S1 Theatre guidelines indicate moist wound-healing products should be used	**P1** Moist wound-healing products are available in the perioperative setting	**O1** Moist wound-healing products are applied as the primary dressing

2. 100% of dressing selections will be based on anticipated volumes of exudate.

Structure	Process	Outcome
S2 Theatre guidelines recommend dressing selection based on anticipated moisture-absorbing requirements of the primary dressing	**P2** Estimated wound fluid loss is evaluated as part of the dressing selection criteria	**O2** Primary dressing applied is of appropriate size and moisture-bearing capacity for the donor site

3. 100 % of primary dressings and reinforcement will be left intact for 24–48 hours postoperatively.

Structure	Process	Outcome
S3 Ward protocols clearly state the need for the primary dressing and reinforcement to be left intact for 24–48 hours postoperatively	**P3** Staff are made aware of the protocol requirements	**O3** All primary donor site dressings and reinforcement are left intact for 24–48 hours postoperatively

Table 7.1 Example of a clinical audit

AUDIT INDICATOR	CRITERIA	AUDIT ACTIVITY	FINDINGS AND COMMENTS	COMPLIANCE Achieved	COMPLIANCE Expected
1	**S1** Theatre guidelines indicate moist wound-healing products should be used	Review procedural guidelines for types of dressings for donor sites	The recommended primary dressings listed were all moist wound-healing products	100%	100%
1	**P1** Moist wound-healing products should be used	Review theatre stores for moist wound-healing products for donor sites	Moist wound-healing products were found to be readily available	100%	100%
1	**O1** Moist wound-healing products are used on all donor sites	Review postoperative patient records for descriptions of types of primary dressings applied	The primary dressings applied were all moist wound-healing products	100%	100%
2	**S2** Theatre guidelines recommend dressing selection based on anticipated moisture-absorbing requirements of the primary dressing	Review theatre guidelines for recommendations to include estimates of wound fluid loss in primary dressing selection	Documented estimates of size and moisture-bearing capacities required of primary dressing were not included in the guidelines	0%	100%
2	**P2** Estimated wound fluid loss is evaluated as part of the dressing selection criteria	Review theatre documentation for evidence of fluid loss estimates	No documented evidence of fluid loss estimates	0%	100%
2	**O2** Type and size of primary dressing is appropriate for the estimated moisture management requirements	Assess frequency of strikethrough by asking nurses on the day of the audit	5 = number with strikethrough 15 = number without strikethrough	75%	100%
3	**S3** Ward protocols clearly state the need for the primary dressing and reinforcement to be left intact for 24–48 hours postoperatively	Review ward-based documentation and practice guidelines	No relevant protocols or documented guidelines were identified	0%	100%
3	**P3** Ward staff are made aware of the protocol requirements	Ask all ward nursing staff rostered on the day of the audit if they know of the protocol requirements	N/A as there were no protocols	N/A	100%
3	**O3** All primary donor site dressings are reinforced for a minimum of 24–48 hours postoperatively	Between 24–48 hours postoperatively, visually inspect all donor sites for the presence of reinforcing	Not all donor sites were left/reinforced for the first 24 hours; some were removed by patients or ward nursing staff	75%	100%

Table 7.1 Example of a clinical audit—cont'd

FACILITY/WARD	CLINICAL AUDITING PROGRAM

AUDIT TOPIC:		Date:
Split-thickness skin graft donor sites: post-harvest management		
Related Standard: JBI 2002 *Best Practice* information sheet 6(2)		

SUMMARY OF AUDIT FINDINGS/COMMENTS AND ACTION PLAN

Indicator 1	
Compliance/Identified problems	Action
100% compliance	No action required

Indicator 2	
Compliance/Identified problems	Action
S2 0% compliance N = compliant N = non compliant	Staff meeting with stakeholders from theatre and ward settings to discuss and clarify the rationale for dressing selection based on estimated moisture management requirements of the primary dressing
P2 0% compliance N = compliant N = non compliant	Reinforcement of the role of documentation as the primary legal avenue for communication of patient care and interventions
O2 75% compliance 15 = no strikethrough 5 = strikethrough	Strikethrough and use of additional reinforcing not found to be as significant a problem as anecdotally suggested. Ward staff to commence 6 weeks of data collection on rates of strikethrough and application of additional reinforcing to clarify the scope of this problem.

Indicator 3	
Compliance/Identified problems	Action
S3 0% compliance **P3** 0% compliance as protocol not yet developed **O3** 0% compliance as protocol not yet developed	Focus group of nursing and medical staff to develop a ward protocol for postoperative management of donor sites, which includes leaving the primary dressing and reinforcing intact for 24–48 hours postoperatively.

CONCLUSIONS AND OUTCOMES OF AUDIT ACTIVITY

The audit indicated that moist wound-healing products were consistently used on all donor sites, achieving 100% compliance with known best practice. The audit also identified that staff were reliant on the availability of up-to-date guidelines to inform practice, and that when such guidelines were missing or incomplete, that practice became variable. This was evident in the lack of structured documentation on assessment of dressing selection and on the requirement to leave primary dressings intact for 24–48 hours postoperatively. The audit results also showed that clinical documentation does not consistently describe the required details of split-thickness skin graft donor sites.
The outcomes of the practice manual review and update will be re-audited in 6 months to measure improvement in outcomes. The current results will be made available to relevant practice areas, with particular focus on the achievement of 100% compliance for audit indicator 1

Table 7.1 Example of a clinical audit—cont'd

make improvements or changes to the area of care if the clinical audit is going to be of any benefit. Because clinical audit aims to compare current practice with an accepted standard, it is useful to identify high-quality standards (such as the JBI *Best Practice* information sheets) and/or develop an audit topic that can be used to compare practice with research evidence such as systematic reviews or randomised controlled trials.

Factors to consider when thinking about a topic for clinical auditing include:

- Do stakeholders have identified concerns with the issue (e.g. complaints)?
- Is there a wide variation in current practice for no obvious beneficial reason?
- Is it an area of high patient risk (e.g. high level of morbidity and/or mortality)?
- Is it an area of high volume (e.g. is it something that is done frequently)?
- Is it an area of high cost (e.g. will you be able to reduce or justify the cost)?
- Is there access to the necessary resources to complete the audit (e.g. time, information, staff)? (Burnett & Winyard 1998, Morrell & Harvey 1999)

In the audit outlined in Table 7.1, the topic selected was postoperative management of split-thickness skin graft donor sites. The care of these wounds was principally a nursing responsibility; thus if practice change was found to be required, the responsibility was clearly within the nursing domain rather than across professional boundaries. Also, donor sites were managed on a single ward, making the audit simple to complete and any required changes easier to negotiate than would have been the case if the audit included multiple wards.

7.9.2 Question development and objectives

Once a topic or practice area has been chosen, it helps to clarify your ideas into a question that others can clearly link to the audit process—the more specific the better. The topic of donor sites was too general to investigate; hence, a specific question was developed from the identified problem. Ideally, the question will clarify who the population of interest is and what the problem is, and may include the standard that practice is being measured against.

In this example, the patients were adults in an acute surgical ward, the problem was that multiple types of dressings were being applied to split-thickness skin donor sites, and there was reliable evidence against which current practice could be reviewed.

Identified problem: Patients with split-thickness skin graft donor site dressings were having frequent dressing changes. The dressing changes were made using numerous product types with the aim of reinforcing or replacing the perioperative dressing when strikethrough occurred.

Specific question: Among adults with postoperative donor site dressings, is current practice in the management of split-thickness skin graft donor site dressings based on the best-available evidence?

Once the question has been established, develop your objectives to maintain the focus of activity. The primary objective of this audit was to ensure that donor site dressing management was congruent with the best available evidence. Objectives are outcome statements that indicate the quality target for the audit. Objectives should be expressed as outcomes statements such as:

Objective: To ensure that postoperative donor site dressings are managed according to the best available evidence.

7.9.3 Identifying best practice

There is no clear consensus about at which point in the audit cycle the evidence should be sought. Some publications suggest that evidence-based standards should be identified or developed once the topic has been selected and before the audit has commenced. Morrell and Harvey (1996) suggest that evidence be used to create standards for implementation prior to auditing. However, others have advocated for a process that audits 'current' practice against an evidence-based standard—effectively establishing the baseline level of compliance between current practice and best practice before making changes to practice. In writing on auditing in clinical guidelines, Hutchinson and Baker (1999) highlight the value of identifying the scope and nature of current clinical practice, and variation within that practice, before introducing new standards. This approach appears to offer the benefit of establishing current compliance before change is introduced.

After the topic for auditing has clearly been stated, identify an evidence source that establishes what best practice is and how it is to be achieved. The evidence can then be used to develop audit indicators. Using a hierarchical approach to choosing evidence sources is a useful strategy for finding high-quality summarised evidence as a priority. This also avoids relying upon individual, unappraised primary research from which to develop measurable audit indicators.

Audit indicators should be based on evidence that they are clinically effective and relevant, and are the basic measure against which practice is compared. Therefore, choosing high-level evidence as the basis of indicator development can facilitate this step. *Audit indicators concisely describe the quality of care to be achieved in definable and measurable terms.* Audit indicators based on best practice evidence provide the most reliable framework for audit activity. In Table 7.1, the audit indicators are based on specific clinical guidelines from a *Best Practice* information sheet developed by the JBI. This demonstrates the link between best evidence and audit indicator development.

7.9.4 Audit indicator development

Indicators are defined as:

> Quantitative statements that are used to measure quality of care. Indicators always include a percentage, ratio or other quantitative way of saying how many patients the expected care should be provided for (National Centre for Clinical Audit 1997).

Indicators must be measurable, observable, relating to only one specific area of practice, and focused on the goal of achieving the best outcome for patients. This will ensure there is a clear means of evaluating whether day-to-day practice is meeting the care standards (Garland & Corfield 2003, Kinn 1995).

Look closely at each audit indicator and decide how data will be collected to determine whether it has been met. It is helpful to identify and develop criteria that need to be met to achieve the indicator in terms of the structure, process and outcome framework. This allows the audit to expand beyond examining outcomes, by including aspects of resource requirements and practical activities that may impact on the outcomes; hence, it is a more encompassing approach.

In order to work effectively within the accepted framework of structure, process and outcome, it is useful to begin with standardised definitions of what these terms mean. The following definitions are established and have been used widely since the mid-1990s:

- *Structure criteria:* these are the resources or what is needed to implement the standard. Structure criteria may include availability of staff and specific equipment or resources such as time required.

- *Process criteria:* these are what needs to be done to implement the care standard—the actions to take and the decisions to make. The process will include aspects such as assessment, evaluation, referral, documentation and specific practical interventions. Examples of process criteria include assessment scales or tools, or care processes to enhance or correct skill and knowledge deficits.
- *Outcome criteria:* these are the anticipated results of the intervention—what you expect to achieve through implementing the care standard. Outcome criteria should contain statements that are measurable, such as percentages or ratios (Kinn 1995; Morrell & Harvey 1996, 1999).

7.9.5 Method

It is common practice to develop an audit protocol, which is used to describe the methods of data collection and analysis, timeline, criteria being evaluated, impact on practice and/or patient outcomes, and to invite participation and/or approval for the project from the appropriate persons within your organisation. Once approval has been obtained, identify and discuss the audit with key stakeholders (clinician groups and/or those with a vested interest in the methods or outcomes of the audit) to gather support for the project. In the accompanying example, the audit was conducted in a tertiary teaching hospital; therefore, permission was sought from the director of nursing and from the service unit involved. Once obtained, a meeting was set up with the clinical nurse consultant and clinicians to explain the audit and obtain their support.

> Data were collected through examination of clinical documentation, including medical records and hospital procedure manuals. The audit was conducted over 4 weeks, and surveyed all patients who underwent procedures that involved a split-thickness skin graft donor site. Twenty patients were identified during the survey period with either a single (n=15) or two or more (n=5) donor sites.

7.9.6 Sampling and data collection

The key issue in audit sampling is to identify the sample size you require so that you can demonstrate either a need for change in practice or that practice is based on the best available evidence. For example, in an audit with a small sample, if the first cases audited were found to be below best practice standards, clearly a problem exists that needs to be addressed, regardless of what the other cases show.

Good audit software will incorporate calculations to recommend an appropriate (statistically significant) sample size. If such software is not available, the sample size should be large enough to give an overall representation of the practice within your facility/area. Be pragmatic! Collecting huge volumes of data looks impressive, but may not be necessary, so collect only what you need in order to address your audit indicators. It is useful to identify whether the entire population can or should be audited; for example, time and financial constraints may dictate choosing a smaller sample. As stated above, even a small sample can be used to detect non-compliance with best practice, and is suggestive that practice improvement is required. It should be noted that with smaller samples it is more difficult to reliably establish actual compliance with best practice if that sample is not representative or lacks statistical power.

Data-collection tools such as checklists or questionnaires can be designed specifically for the audit or can be adapted from pre-existing collection tools (such as the example at the end of this chapter). When collecting and recording the data, be considerate of basic research principles such as ethical considerations and confidentiality. Collecting data is the most visible part of the audit process.

In our example, audit data were collected through a short-answer/closed-ended questionnaire. The findings of the questions were compiled into the audit outline as percentages of expected and achieved outcomes. The results showed that the primary dressings applied in the perioperative setting were either Duoderm or Kaltostat, both of which are moist wound-healing products. Of the 17 donor sites, 15 required further reinforcement or change of dressing, and two did not require any additional intervention. A total of 114 extra items were used, including combines, crepe bandages, Duoderm, Hypafix and Chux.

The reasons for reinforcement or replacement of the dressings were:
- leakage of exudates from the primary dressing
- primary dressing removed by the patient
- Kaltostat changed to Duoderm to decrease risk of adherence to the wound bed
- *Pseudomonas* infection present in the wound.

7.9.7 Data analysis and evaluation

Data analysis involves looking at the numbers to identify the percentage or degree of compliance between practice and the audit criteria. Good audit software will automatically generate figures, graphs or tables that show the level of compliance per criterion and these can be copied into an audit report or presentation. However, a second and often more challenging aspect of data analysis is to evaluate why current practice did or did not meet the expected standards.

It can be useful at this stage to call a meeting of the project team, or stakeholders, and present the audit results for discussion. Ideally, discussion will centre on identifying the potential barriers to achieving compliance, the types of strategies that can practicably be implemented to facilitate compliance, the key persons to involve in each strategy, and the types of resources they might need in order to implement best practice. Discussion should also focus on a timeline that describes the activity to be undertaken and maps out the resources needed to address the identified barriers and the key people involved.

Evaluation of the audit data in our example found that current practice was not consistent with best practice—of the 17 donor sites, 15 had dressing changes or additions, with a total of 114 additional dressing products. While the primary dressings were moist wound-healing products, the number of additional products being used, and the reports of strikethrough as a cause of dressing changes/reinforcement, suggest that perioperative dressing selection and ward-based protocols could be improved to increase the use of primary dressings with additional moisture-bearing capacities, and to increase the use of additional reinforcing rather than replacement. Also, the range of additional dressing products being applied could be reduced, promoting greater consistency in patient care delivery and potentially reducing costs.

7.9.8 Feedback

There are a range of views on what to do once you have collected the audit data. Some sources suggest you should evaluate the data and return to the key stakeholders with that information for them to discuss, and potentially develop further action frameworks (Morrell & Harvey 1999). However, this approach relies on the use of an audit group who will assist in the audit process and in establishing an action plan once the data have been collected and evaluated. These resources are not always available and therefore it is useful to make a list of potential methods for communicating the audit results where they will be most effective. Consider avenues of personal one-to-one communication in addition to group presentations, and consider written communication through available resources.

The value of feedback of audit results is that it can enhance a sense of ownership. Through feedback, health professionals get to see the effects of their practice and, although potentially a threatening scenario, it can be highly motivating. Feedback should be carefully considered and structured in order to gain maximum benefit; that is, to increase the likelihood that practice change will continue and be sustained. Poorly constructed feedback, such as criticism that is not constructive or well presented, may undo previous good work at stimulating practice improvement.

7.9.9 Implementing best practice (standard/s)

If the above approach to the audit cycle has been followed, you are now well positioned to implement an EBP change-management strategy. Baseline data have been collected that compare current practice with a best practice standard, the data have been analysed, the barriers to compliance, people and resources required to improve practice have been identified, and the key stakeholders have been involved throughout, and are aware of the need for practice change.

This cycle presents a compelling case for changing current practice. The evaluation of barriers, resources and strategies provides the framework for implementation of new evidence-based standards, and this may be further facilitated by good audit software that tracks timelines and facilitates the getting of research (best practice) into practice.

Implementation, or knowledge utilisation, has developed its own body of science and theory; it is outside the scope of this chapter to represent that body of knowledge. Reading widely on the topic of 'knowledge utilisation' or 'implementation' will give a broad perspective on strategies that can be used to facilitate implementation of best practice.

Factors that may impact on the effectiveness of the implementation process may include the level of openness with which the audit data and practice-change strategies are communicated. For effective implementation it is important that staff members feel a 'sense of ownership'. Exchanging information and being open to feedback from colleagues will raise awareness of your audit activity, encourage communication and improve the adoption rate of new practice.

Time is always a factor in healthcare. More (or less) time may be required between implementation of the standard/s and any subsequent re-auditing, depending on the complexity of the topic and/or the size of the organisation. Some topics are organisational key performance indicators and subject to ongoing audit. (This was not the case in the audit scenario in this chapter. In our example, the *Best Practice* standards were widely circulated and all staff had the opportunity to read and gain familiarity with the recommendations for practice.) A basic rule of thumb for establishing when to re-audit is to allow enough time for implementation of best practice, without allowing so much time that the project loses momentum.

7.9.10 Re-auditing

The first issue to consider is whether, and with what frequency, a topic warrants re-auditing. It is sometimes difficult to establish the frequency with which to re-audit topics that are not considered high organisational priorities. Some aspects of practice require continuous audit; these include quality and safety standards, incident monitoring, and key performance indicator outcomes.

The minimum duration between audit and re-audit should be the time frame required for all initial indicators to be implemented. The time frame should also include consideration of staff workloads, other concurrent activities, key stakeholder interest and momentum. Another consideration is that if the audit criteria were developed from evidence or guidelines that are updated regularly, the timing of the updates, particularly if there is a clinically significant change in the update, can be used as a guide. A follow-up audit will then provide useful data that identifies where practice change has been achieved as well as those areas that require further work, thus indicating the sustainability of changes that have been effected.

7.10 Conclusion

An expected outcome of patient assessment and care planning is that nurses make decisions about patient care that result in changes to practice. When decisions to change practice are made, it is important to establish that the changes have been implemented correctly and that the expected outcomes are being achieved. Determining whether changes in care provision have actually influenced patient outcomes is a crucial step in the evidence-based cycle (Flemming & Fenton 2002) and can be undertaken through clinical audit. Moreover, evaluation through clinical audit can take place either before or following the initiation of best practice. While clinical audit is most often cited as a tool for use in the evaluation phase of the evidence-based cycle, it is in fact an excellent tool for encouraging the implementation of best practice and generating an evidence-based culture (Shakib 2002). Through continually reviewing the delivery of care and taking action to improve it when deficiencies are identified (Kinn 1995:35), clinical audit is used to develop and refine healthcare practices (Morrell & Harvey 1999).

This chapter reviewed the concept of clinical audit and its place in EBP. An example drawn from practice has been provided as a template to audit and other useful resources have been identified. Clinical audits require a structured approach to their design and implementation. Attention should be given to institutional approval, where appropriate a multidisciplinary approach, and in all cases careful planning and rigorous implementation. All of the material provided in this chapter is designed to assist clinicians to more confidently undertake audit. In this way, audit can become a routine part of healthcare, thus facilitating a process of continuous quality improvement and increased standards of care.

7.11 DISCUSSION QUESTIONS

1. Consider your own area of practice. What topic/s do you think would be suitable for clinical audit?
2. What factors should influence the decision to audit a particular issue or topic?
3. What role does clinical audit play in promoting EBP?
4. What is the relationship between EBP and quality improvement?
5. What skills are needed to undertake a clinical audit?
6. What barriers might impact on your ability to conduct a clinical audit? How might these be overcome?

7.12 **References**

Balogh R 1996 Exploring the links between audit and the research process. *Nurse Researcher* 3(3):5–16.

Borbasi S, Jackson D, Langford R W 2008 *Navigating the maze of nursing research: an interactive learning adventure, 2nd edn.* Elsevier, Sydney.

Burnett A, Winyard G 1998 Clinical audit at the heart of clinical effectiveness. *Journal of Quality in Clinical Practice* 18(1):3–19.

Clinical Audit Central Office, University Hospitals Bristol NHS Foundation Trust 2005 *How to apply ethics to clinical audit.* Available: www.uhbristol.nhs.uk/healthcare-professionals/clinical-audit/how-to-guides.html 16 May 2009.

Closs S, Cheater P 1996 Audit or research – what is the difference? *Journal of Clinical Nursing* 5(4):249–56.

Department of Health 1993 *Clinical audit – meeting and improving standards in health care.* Department of Health, London.

Flemming K, Fenton M 2002 Making sense of research evidence to inform decision making. In: Thompson C, Dowding D (eds) *Clinical decision-making and judgement in nursing.* Churchill Livingstone, Edinburgh, pp 109–29.

Garland G, Corfield F 2003 Audit. In: Hamer S, Collinson G (eds) *Achieving evidence-based practice, 2nd edn.* Bailliere Tindall, London, pp 129–49.

Gaston C 2003 *Governance in the South Australian public health system: briefing paper no 4. Generational Health Review.* Department of Human Services, Adelaide.

Joanna Briggs Institute (JBI) 2002 Split-thickness skin graft donor sites: post-harvest management. *Best Practice* information sheet 6(2).

Hutchinson A, Baker R 1999 *Making use of guidelines in clinical practice.* Radcliff Medical Press, Oxon.

Kinn S 1995 Clinical audit: a tool for practice. *Nursing Standard* 9(15):35–6.

Mason A 2002 The emerging role of clinical audits. *Clinical Medicine* 2(4):294–6.

Mead D, Moseley L 1996 Research-based measurement tools in the audit process: issues of use, validity and reliability. *Nurse Researcher* 3(3):17–34.

Morrell C, Harvey G 1996 Clinical audit. *Nursing Standard* 10(17):38–44.

Morrell C, Harvey G 1999 *The clinical audit handbook.* Bailliere Tindall, London.

Morrell C, Harvey G, Kitson A L 1995 *The reality of practitioner-based quality improvement, Report no. 14.* National Institute for Nursing, Oxford.

National Centre for Clinical Audit 1997 *Key points from audit literature related to criteria for clinical audit.* National Centre for Clinical Audit, London.

National Institute for Clinical Excellence (NICE) 2002 *Principles for best practice in clinical audit.* Radcliffe Medical Press, Oxford. Available: www.nice.org.uk/media/796/23/BestPracticeClinicalAudit.pdf 16 May 2009.

National Institute for Health and Clinical Excellence (NICE). Available: www.nice.org.uk 14 May 2009.

Perry L 2007 Implementing best evidence in clinical practice. In: Craig J V, Smyth R L (eds) *The evidence-based practice manual for nurses, 2nd edn.* Churchill Livingstone, Edinburgh, pp 267–304.

Scally G, Donaldson L J 1998 Clinical governance and the drive for quality improvement in the new NHS in England. *British Medical Journal* 317(7150):61–5.

Scott P V 2000 Differentiating between audit and research: clinical audit is research. 320(7236):713.

Shakib S 2003 Auditmaker: a generic tool for clinical audit. Available: www.auditmaker.org 8 Aug 2009.

Thomas B 1999 Research and audit in effective health services. *Nursing Standard* 13(33): 40–2.

Thompson C, Learmonth M 2002 How can we develop an evidence-based culture? In: Craig J V, Smyth R L (eds) *The evidence-based practice manual for nurses.* Churchill Livingstone, Edinburgh, pp 211–39.

University Hospitals Bristol, NHS. *How to guides.* Available: www.uhbristol.nhs.uk/
healthcare-professionals/clinical-audit/how-to-guides.html 21 May 2009.
Walshe K, Spurgeon P 1997 *Clinical audit assessment framework handbook series 24.* Health
Services Management Centre, University of Birmingham, Birmingham.
World Health Organisation 1983 *The principles of quality assurance* (report on a WHO meeting).
World Health Organisation, Copenhagen.

CHAPTER 8

Undertaking a program evaluation

Elizabeth Manias

8.1 Learning objectives

After reading this chapter, you should be able to:

1. define important components of a program, including the goal, outcome, strategy, performance indicator and performance measure
2. describe the purpose of the five types of program evaluation: proactive, clarificative, interactive, monitoring, and impact, and
3. determine the type of program to be undertaken in terms of the questions being asked about the program and the timing of its delivery.

8.2 Introduction

Quite reasonably, the use of evidence-based practice (EBP) and provision of quality care means that nurses need to demonstrate how their nursing-care activities work and to give rationales for why they work. Completing a program evaluation provides a formalised way of addressing this need. This chapter provides an overview of the processes involved in a program evaluation. We consider definitions of essential terms used in program evaluations and then examine five forms of evaluation that underpin evaluative activities: proactive, clarificative, interactive, monitoring, and impact. Finally, we provide case studies from the health literature that illustrate how these forms of evaluation are used.

8.3 Definitions

Program evaluation involves the process of conducting a systematic appraisal of a particular activity for the purpose of generating knowledge and planning future strategies. Another term that is sometimes used for program evaluation is outcomes research. A number of definitions of program evaluation exist. Green (1990), who refers to the importance of benchmarking, defines program evaluation as comparing an activity of interest with a standard of acceptability. This definition is useful because it includes the process, impact and outcomes that can be examined, and facilitates a range of standards of acceptability.

Evaluation must be congruent with the goals and objectives of the program activity and the measurement of these activities needs to be appropriate. Evaluation is also a continuous process of asking questions, thinking about the responses, and reviewing the planned strategy and activity (Fleming & Parker 2007).

Several other parameters are important in undertaking a program evaluation; they include the program's goals, outcomes, strategies, objectives, performance indicators and performance measures. These parameters are explained in Table 8.1. These terms are interpreted in different ways. Government organisations and funding bodies often use their own specific definitions of these terms, and it is important to use the definitions provided by these instrumentalities to make sure that particular components are addressed (Department of Health and Aged Care 2001).

8.4 Forms of program evaluation

Program evaluation is classified according to the purpose of the intended activities. There are five forms of evaluation that underpin the various roles of evaluative activities: proactive, clarificative, interactive, monitoring, and impact (Owen & Rogers 1999). Table 8.2 shows the basic elements of each form, including the purpose, focus and timing for program delivery. It is important to note that within a program evaluation one might also use aspects of clinical audit or evidence-based guideline review, so it is advisable to make yourself familiar with the contents of Chapters 4 and 7.

8.4.1 Proactive evaluation

Proactive evaluation takes place before the program commences. Its purpose is to provide evidence of what is known about the issue, and to use this information in deciding how to develop a program. It also provides managers with details on how an organisation needs to change to improve its effectiveness (Owen & Rogers 1999, Scheirer 1998).

Some of the characteristic questions of this form include:
- Is there a need for the program at all?
- What are the best practice guidelines in this area?
- What research is currently available about this problem?

Three main approaches are used with this form of analysis: needs assessment, review of available literature, and review of best practice guidelines. A needs assessment addresses

Term	Meaning
Goal	The aim that the initiative seeks to achieve in general
Outcome	The changes in attitude, behaviour, health condition or status that the initiative seeks to achieve. It also concerns learning outcomes in relation to process, knowledge and skills
Strategy	The plan used to achieve the desired outcomes
Objective	The specific targets that need to be accomplished in an effort to achieve the outcomes
Performance indicator	The responses or measured changes in attitude, behaviour, health condition or status that indicate progress towards objectives and outcomes
Performance measure	The way in which changes in attitude, behaviour, health condition or status will be measured

Table 8.1 Parameters in a program evaluation

	Proactive	**Clarificative**	**Interactive**	**Monitoring**	**Impact**
Purpose of evaluation	Synthesis of program	Provide explanation	Improvement	Justification, refinement	Justification, accountability
Focus	Context of program	Development of program	Development of program	Delivery and outcome of program	Delivery and outcome of program
Timing on program delivery	Before	During	During	During	After

Table 8.2 Evaluation forms: Purpose, focus and timing
Adapted from Owen & Rogers 1999

the problems or conditions of a particular community or organisation that should be included in future planning. It usually occurs when individuals are concerned about the present situation and type of service delivery. This approach provides valuable information about the initiatives that could be implemented to improve the situation in the future. A needs assessment is helpful in setting priorities for healthcare and allocating scarce resources. In addressing a need for a particular program, evaluators are concerned about differences between the current and desired situations, thereby establishing discrepancies. Reasons are sought for these discrepancies and decisions can be made about which needs should be given priority for action (Roth 1990).

A review of available literature involves collating what is known about the area of inquiry. It includes an examination of research publications and systematic reviews that may have already been completed on the area of interest. Most importantly, it considers how previous research has been applied to the practice setting. After the current state of research work is described and critiqued, the review should give some indication of the gaps in knowledge on the topic.

A review of best practice guidelines requires selecting and examining exemplary practice in the area; such an approach enables the creation of benchmarks. Benchmarking has become very prominent over recent times, as organisations such as hospitals, universities and government bodies model their activities against known leaders in their field. In establishing benchmarks, it is important to identify the area of best practice, and consider whether this practice applies to the organisation. Evaluators determine how the practice is performed, and how well it is carried out relative to the best markers. After comparisons are made, it is important for managers to determine how they want the organisation to perform, relative to exemplary practice.

Data collection methods employed in proactive evaluation involve review of documents and databases, the Delphi technique, strategic planning meetings and focus groups. Examples of documents and databases that may be reviewed include hospital data such as morbidity, mortality and length of hospital stay (Centers for Disease Control and Prevention 1999). The Delphi technique requires individuals to work independently and to pool their written ideas about a particular issue. Each individual is given a list of the collected ideas, which are formatted into a set of scaled items, and asked to assess their relative importance and relevance. Strategic planning meetings are events designed to provide direction for a projected program. Individuals involved in delivering the program collaborate to consider barriers and facilitators to achieving certain activities, what they have achieved and what they wish to achieve in the future. The focus group is a method that aims to collect information from a selected group of people. While the goal of the Delphi technique is to achieve consensus, the desired outcome of focus groups is to obtain a range of views.

The following case studies are provided to highlight how proactive evaluation uses literature review and evidence-based guideline review to inform the program of work to be implemented (see Ch 4 on developing evidence-based guidelines).

CASE STUDY: Review of available literature and best practice guidelines

Bucknall et al (2001) examined best practice guidelines for acute pain against past research on pain. The paper evaluated the implications of the National Health and Medical Research Council (NHMRC) acute pain guidelines on nursing practice, and addressed the inadequacies of current implementation policies of hospitals. The authors argued that the NHMRC pain management guidelines failed to decrease patients' pain because healthcare professionals, organisations and researchers largely ignored the impact of contextual issues on clinical decision making. Contextual issues included patient involvement and control, nurses' pain assessment and management skills, multidisciplinary collaboration, organisational management, educational needs and evaluation of pain-management effectiveness. The authors recommended that future pain management programs should consider acknowledging contextual issues in their development and implementation.

CASE STUDY: Review of available literature and hospital protocols

With increasing technology and medication complexity, hospital policies and protocols are helpful in supporting nurses to integrate new knowledge into practice and to guide effective decision making. Manias et al (2005) examined how newly graduated nurses used hospital protocols in their medication management activities. While some protocols were developed from evidence-based guidelines, such as checking the patient's identity before medication administration, others were derived from what was considered to be good practice in the hospital, such as double checking of opiate medications. Newly graduated nurses were observed and interviewed on how they carried out various medication protocols. These protocols included: checking the patient's identity before administering medication; double checking the administration of parenteral or opioid medications with another nurse; checking the identity band of the patient against the identity label on the medication order; writing or initiating medication incident reports if a medication error occurred; following up of unclear medication orders with an experienced doctor or nurse; checking unknown medications using written medication resources; and observing patients actually consuming oral medications. Some protocols were observed to be followed according to expected recommendations. There were 34 situations observed where nurses were confronted with an unclear medication order, and in all of these situations they sought advice from an experienced doctor or nurse. Nurses observed patients taking oral medications in 90% of situations (118/131), and in 80% of situations they administered parenteral or opioid medications using a double checking procedure with other nurses (24/30). They were also observed to follow up on unknown medications in 86% of situations (12/14). There were two medication errors associated with medication administration; however, these were not documented as medication incidents. In addition, patients' identity labels were only checked in 27% of situations (48/175). The study demonstrated that evaluation of protocol adherence can be a useful means of determining the extent to which nurses provide safe medication management.

8.4.2 Clarificative evaluation

Clarificative evaluation is to examine the underlying structure, rationale and function of a program. It focuses on the internal components of a program rather than the way in which the program is implemented. The need for clarification may occur when there are conflicts over components of a program's design. Individuals may also require further details about how the program activities link with intended outcomes (Owen & Rogers 1999).

Characteristic questions associated with this form of evaluation include:
- What is the rationale for this program?
- What are the intended outcomes for this program?
- What structures need to be changed to ensure that intended outcomes are achieved?

Two main approaches are used in this form of evaluation: program logic development and accreditation (Owen & Rogers 1999). Program logic development involves examining available documentation and conducting interviews with relevant stakeholders to construct an overview of what the program is intended to do. It also considers how the current program could be changed to address the intended outcomes.

Accreditation determines the worth of a particular program. In health and education arenas, it involves the process of certifying that an organisation can deliver the program activity over a particular time period. This approach provides consumers with the confidence of knowing that accredited programs are of an acceptable quality.

Data collected for clarificative evaluation usually include document analysis, interviews and observations. Document sources could involve policy statements, memoranda, hospital reports, legislation, and meeting agenda and minutes. In conducting interviews and observations, the goal is to identify the most critical elements of a program between members of the evaluation team and key program staff. The views of stakeholders are also sought and compared to the elements identified in interactions between program and evaluation staff. Decisions can then be made about how the program can be implemented.

The following case studies are provided to highlight how clarificative evaluation examines underlying structure, rationale and function to determine whether the design of the program met the needs of the program participants.

> ### CASE STUDY: Program logic development 1
>
> Manias et al (2000) described the benefits of combining objective and naturalistic methods when undertaking a formative evaluation of a computer-assisted learning program in pharmacology for nursing students. During the design and development phases, the pharmacology program was evaluated using observation of student pairs, student questionnaires and student focus group interviews. The combination of evaluation methods enabled complex issues underlying the program effectiveness to be addressed.

> ### CASE STUDY: Program logic development 2
>
> Ellis and Hogard (2003) evaluated a pilot scheme for clinical facilitators in acute medical and surgical wards. The clinical facilitators were employed to address two issues: i) the nursing skills demonstrated by newly graduated nurses, and ii) concerns about supervision in clinical placement. The purpose of the clinical facilitators was to enhance undergraduate nurses' competence on clinical placement. Evaluation involved a three-phase approach covering outcomes, process and multiple stakeholder views. The work of clinical facilitators was evaluated using interviews, focus groups and questionnaires with students, clinical staff and university staff. While clinical facilitators were evaluated in a positive way, concerns were raised about communication. University staff also tended to rate the clinical facilitators less favourably than did students and clinical staff.

8.4.3 Interactive evaluation

Interactive evaluation examines the delivery and implementation of a program. Because this form of evaluation is particularly important for program activities that are constantly changing, it has a strong element of improving processes (see Ch 7 on undertaking a clinical audit). Individuals are also given an opportunity to better understand how and why a program functions in certain ways. This form of evaluation does not focus on the outcomes or the end products of the program. Key stakeholders are more interested in undertaking an evaluation that supports change and improvement (Owen & Rogers 1999).

Characteristic questions associated with this form of evaluation include:
- How is the delivery of the program working?
- What is the program attempting to achieve?
- How can the delivery be changed to make program delivery more effective?
- How can the organisation be changed to make program delivery more effective?

Approaches used in interactive evaluation involve responsive evaluation, action research (discussed in Ch 7) and quality review. Responsive evaluation involves a detailed documentation of the implementation of a program. It takes into account the views and values of various stakeholders including the providers and consumers (Guba & Lincoln 1981, 1989; Patton 2002). An evaluation is considered responsive if it is orientated more towards the activities of the program rather than its purpose or outcomes.

Action research involves an intensive and reflective process of determining whether the various methods of program delivery are making a difference. It requires the evaluator to go into the environment and work with individuals as co-researchers or co-evaluators, in an attempt to find solutions to problems. Solutions to problems are collaboratively decided upon, carried out and examined through reflection (Wadsworth 1997). Action research involves a cyclical, systematic process of planning, acting, observing and reflecting, which subsequently leads to a revised plan, and further acting, observing and reflecting (Reason & Bradbury 2007).

Quality reviews take place within the organisation delivering the program. Individuals within the organisation evaluate their processes and make changes depending on initiatives developed at the wider organisational level (see Ch 7). Individuals delivering the program usually carry out quality reviews—expertise through experienced evaluators is not usually available (Colton 1997, Owen & Rogers 1999).

Data-collection methods for responsive evaluation and quality reviews involve reflective journalling, collaborative meetings and strategic-planning workshops. Methods commonly used in action research include participant observation, interviews and reflective journalling (Greenwood & Levin 2006). Participants may include consumers or providers of program initiatives.

The following case studies are provided to highlight how interactive evaluation uses quality review and action research to examine and determine the success of the delivery and implementation of a program.

CASE STUDY: Quality review

Manias and Aitken (2003) described the development, implementation and evaluation of a new critical-care nursing curriculum. They examined lecturers' and clinical educators' views, and explored students' perspectives of the old curriculum compared with the new curriculum. Three data-collection methods were used for this quality review. Comprehensive and reflective notes were kept of meetings conducted during the development and implementation of the curriculum. Focus group interviews were conducted with students before and during the introduction of the new curriculum. Anonymous quality of teaching surveys, which were distributed by a centralised university process, were also completed by two groups of critical-care nursing students: one before and the other following the introduction of the new curriculum. Evaluation of the development and implementation enabled the investigators to further refine the curriculum to address the challenging and competing needs of clinical educators, clinical nurses, lecturers, students and university management.

CASE STUDY: Action research

Dickinson et al (2008) sought to improve the mealtime experience of older people requiring complex medical and nursing care in hospital. The investigators collaborated with nurses working in the ward in effort to gauge an understanding of the practice setting, the concern about poor nutrition and the culture of the environment. All nurses in the ward were regarded as collaborators in the research to facilitate learning and bring about critical reflection in a supportive and enabling way. Observations were conducted of mealtimes to determine the factors that impacted on patient care. Focus groups were also undertaken with a variety of health professionals to capture different perspectives about mealtimes and mealtime care. Health professionals included in the focus groups were: nutrition assistants, nursing staff, occupational therapists and physiotherapists. Photographs taken during mealtimes on the ward were used to stimulate discussion among group participants. Patients participated in individual interviews to obtain their views about the mealtime experience. Once the mealtime experience had been examined from different perspectives, the research team worked with all staff to engage in role modelling of good practice and to identify solutions for barriers associated with mealtime care. Targeted educational sessions were implemented; these focused on the use of nutrition assessment tools and eating equipment. Evaluations for change were assessed through the recording of field notes and reflective diaries.

The findings of Dickinson et al (2008) showed that mealtime care had initially operated in a ritualised manner with little consideration of the individual nutritional needs of patients. Assisting patients at mealtimes was an activity undertaken by unqualified assistants while qualified nurses attended to other priorities of care such as medication administration and completion of paperwork. There was no systematic screening of the nutritional needs or preferences of patients, and health professionals were largely not involved in decision making about food choices or food portion size. After health professionals reflected on the problems relating to patients' mealtimes, major changes in practice occurred. Nurses took the time to find out what patients would like to eat, and nutritional assessment and monitoring became more evident. Time was taken during handover, ward meetings and conversations with patients and family to discuss patients' mealtime needs.

8.4.4 Monitoring evaluation

Monitoring evaluation is applied when a program is established. Individuals are usually familiar with the goals and outcomes, and have begun to implement the program. The need to undertake this form of evaluation arises from managers who wish to determine the success of a program, analyse its effectiveness and analyse efficiencies as the program is implemented (Grembowski 2001, Hulscher et al 1999, Owen & Rogers 1999).

Characteristic questions associated with this form of evaluation include:
- How is the program reaching its target population?
- What are the costs of implementing the program and how do these compare with expectations?
- Can the program be changed to make it more effective?
- Can the program be changed to make it more efficient?
- How is implementation of the program meeting anticipated benchmarks?

Approaches used in this form of evaluation involve component analysis, devolved performance assessment and systems analysis (Owen & Rogers 1999). Component analysis requires a systematic examination of a particular aspect of the program, which is then compared to the overall goals of the organisation and the program. In deciding upon which component to investigate, managers may consider selecting a poorly running, new or expensive intervention.

Devolved performance assessment is the process whereby individuals who work in specific departments of an organisation set up evaluation procedures that report regularly to managers about their progress. This approach involves assessing the performance of all components of a program on a regular basis. Senior managers receive these assessments and make judgments about how the components contribute to the overall mission of the organisation and the goals of the program.

Systems analysis involves the central managers setting up uniform evaluation procedures that are used by all departments of the organisation. This type of approach is centrally specified and disseminated for implementation to a large number of sites. An example may include the Course Experience Questionnaire that is sent out by the Department of Education, Science and Technology to every Australian graduating university student.

Data-collection methods involve examining particular indicators, which allow judgments to be made about the quality and effectiveness of a program. Indicators are used to compare a program's trends over time, and to compare the performance of a program against an acceptable set of standards. They are also valuable for comparing the implementation of the same program at different sites. Indicators must give details about the program's appropriateness, efficiency and effectiveness. In other words, indicators should provide information about how the program's objectives match with community and government expectations, the relative cost of achieving a positive impact from the program, and how the program's objectives compare with its outcomes (Owen 2006). An example of an efficiency indicator is the ratio of the number of patients in a cardiac rehabilitation program related to the cost of running such a program. Using the same example, an effectiveness indicator could involve the ratio of the number of patients in a cardiac rehabilitation program who do not experience a myocardial infarction in a given time, versus the number who have enrolled in the program.

The following case study provides an example of how component analysis is used to compare one aspect of a program to the overall goals of the organisation and the program, and how doing so can result in minor changes being made to the program that result in better patient outcomes.

CASE STUDY: Component analysis

The Office of Statewide Health Planning and Development in California collects and disseminates financial and clinical data from licensed health facilities (Joint Commission on Accreditation of Healthcare Organizations & National Pharmaceutical Council 2003). Managers and healthcare professionals at the University of California Medical Center expanded the mandated data collection to include data obtained from pain assessment interviews and chart audits. While these data were maintained for internal use, the hospital obtained this information to provide quarterly performance information that could be used to determine trends and track effectiveness. For instance, in one particular initiative, the charts of 433 patients were reviewed. It was found that a hospital-specific documentation standard was met in only 39% of charts. A structural barrier relating to the forms used was identified, which was easily corrected to improve the score. Following this change, 217 patients were interviewed and 92% reported that pain relief action was taken within 20 minutes of their communication of pain.

8.4.5 Impact evaluation

Impact evaluation involves an analysis of an established program. While a major intent of impact evaluation is to determine outcomes, it may also examine how the program is implemented. Following the conduct of impact evaluation, a decision is made about whether the program made a difference to the groups receiving it, or whether one program was better than another. Judgments can then be made about whether to continue with an activity or to change it in some way. Impact evaluation is retrospective because it is undertaken on programs that have had sufficient time to create an effect (Grembowski 2001, Owen & Rogers 1999).

Characteristic issues of this form of evaluation include:
- How cost-effective has the program been?
- To what extent have the anticipated goals been met?
- Were any unintended outcomes apparent?
- How adequately has the program served individuals' needs?

There are four main approaches to this form of evaluation: objectives-based evaluation, process–outcomes analysis, needs-based assessment, and performance audit (Owen & Rogers 1999). An objectives-based evaluation requires examining the extent to which the stated objectives of the program have been achieved. In identifying the objectives of the program, a variety of sources may be used, including policy documents, position statements for the role of different healthcare professionals and program statements. Interviews with relevant stakeholders should be undertaken, and may include nursing students, nurses, patients and representatives of health-regulating and professional bodies (Brandon 1999). If using instrument tools to determine the transfer of program objectives into outcomes, it is important to ensure that they have been validated. If suitable instruments are not available, evaluators may need to develop new measures that accurately reflect the intention of the program.

A process–outcomes analysis involves scrutinising the way in which a program is implemented. In this approach, the focus is on how a program is put into practice and the effect that this has on the intentions of the program. Observational techniques are the best way in which to undertake this approach.

A needs-based assessment has already been described and involves the degree to which the program meets the needs of the individuals using it. The assumption made in considering this approach is that the goals of the program may not necessarily reflect the consumers' needs. A needs-based approach adopts an external standard of reference to determine a program's worth.

Finally, a performance audit involves analysing if the program actually produces expected benefits, and the cost associated with these benefits. The basic premises of a performance audit are that healthcare resources are scarce, there are insufficient resources to satisfy all wants, resources have different uses, and people have different wants (Elixhauser et al 1998, Grembowski 2001, Reid 2000, Rice 2007). The challenge involves deciding how to allocate scarce resources to satisfy individual wants. There are four ways in which cost can be evaluated in economic terms (see Table 8.3). It is important to note that economic evaluation determines the cost of a program as well as its outcomes. Organisational factors can change the effectiveness of programs. For example, cost-effectiveness varies depending on the relative cost of the clinical staff involved in implementing the program (Thorogood & Coombes 2006). Nurses and other healthcare professionals are often used in evaluation endeavours because they are cheaper to employ than doctors.

Cost-effectiveness also varies according to the risk level of populations involved. Thus, in some cases, interventions directed at patients at high risk are more efficient than those

Type of economic evaluation	Characteristics
Cost-effectiveness analysis (CEA)	This type of analysis allows judgments to be made about the relative efficiency of alternative ways of achieving a desired benefit. A program is efficient if no other program is as effective at a lower cost.
Cost–benefit analysis (CBA)	The program is considered to have value when its benefit is equal to or exceeds its costs, or the ratio of benefits to costs is equal to or greater than 1.0 for a particular program. Alternatively, the cost–benefit ratio of one program is equal to or exceeds the cost–benefit ratio of another program.
Cost-minimisation analysis (CMA)	Two programs are considered to have identical outcomes, and the goal of analysis is to determine which program has the lower cost.
Cost–utility analysis (CUA)	The outcomes of two programs are weighted by their value or quality, which is determined by a common measure such as 'quality-adjusted years'. The goal of analysis is to determine which program has the most quality-adjusted life years at lower cost.

Table 8.3 Performance audit describing four ways of economic evaluation of programs
Adapted from Grembowski 2001

directed at patients at a relative low risk. In the healthcare sector, economic efficiency refers to the ability to maximise health outcomes with a given amount of resources. In determining outcomes in economic terms, the objectives of the program are reduced to measures of efficiency. This approach advocates the more efficient the program, the more worthy it is. Typically, most impact evaluations consider cost implications together with other health-related outcomes, such as quality of life, re-admission to hospital and functional ability. Table 8.3 describes the different ways in which the economic attributes of a program can be evaluated.

Impact evaluation involves the use of experimental or descriptive–exploratory research designs to test the effectiveness of a program. Examples include quasi-experimental comparative, controlled studies, randomised controlled trials (RCTs), and qualitative studies using observations and interviews. Validated instruments are used to test the effectiveness of a program. Analyses of policy documents and program statements are also conducted. For process–product studies, observations and interviews are undertaken with program providers and consumers to determine whether the goals of the program have been met. The results of the evaluation are presented to the policy makers who will make rational decisions about its benefits.

The following case studies provide examples of how process–product studies and objectives-based evaluation and performance audit can inform improvements and changes to programs.

CASE STUDY: Process–product study

Manias and Bullock (2002) examined the effectiveness of pharmacology education in undergraduate and graduate nursing programs in preparing graduate nurses for clinical practice. The study was undertaken by two university academics who had no formal collaborative links with the participating clinical nurses or hospitals. Six focus group interviews were conducted with clinical nurses at two metropolitan and two regional hospitals, in which information was sought about their perceptions and experiences of graduate nurses' pharmacology knowledge. Four themes were identified. Participants indicated that graduate nurses had enormous deficits in their pharmacology knowledge. There was an unstructured approach with addressing the continuing education needs of graduate nurses. Participants valued the importance of theoretical and clinical principles of pharmacology knowledge for safe nursing practice. Finally, they believed university undergraduate nursing education should instil a greater sense of responsibility and accountability among students in their monitoring and administering of medications. The investigators concluded that current teaching and learning opportunities at the undergraduate and graduate levels were inadequate in developing and enhancing nurses' pharmacology knowledge.

CASE STUDY: Objectives-based evaluation and performance audit

Dornan et al (2006) examined how medical students' evaluation of their clinical learning environment, process and outcome correlated with their summative assessment results. The study was conducted in the third year of a 5-year medical degree with students undertaking an objectives-based clinical curriculum. Students evaluated what they learned and the manner in which they learned the material using a validated web-based scale. Their evaluations were examined according to four areas: real patient learning, curriculum coverage, quality of instruction, and conditions for learning. Evaluations of the environment, process and outcome correlated with students' assessments in two areas: real patient learning and curriculum coverage. The study showed that a curriculum involving clear learning objectives, supported by problem-based learning tutorials, hospital seminars and skills laboratory training, had a positive effect on their learning. In addition, an emphasis on real patient learning provided students with rich clinical experiences and impacted on students' clinical competence.

CASE STUDY: Performance audit as part of an intervention

Thomas et al (2007) conducted an RCT to assess the effects of a registry-generated audit, feedback, and patient-reminder-system intervention on diabetes care. Participants comprised 78 physicians caring for 483 patients with diabetes in hospital clinics. Physicians who were randomised to the intervention group received two 1-hour education sessions on the use of a computerised diabetes registry that provided details of all their patients with diabetes. The registry gave information on quarterly performance audits, feedback and written reports identifying patients who were not compliant with treatment recommendations. This group also had letters recommending pathology tests sent out automatically to patients who had not had haemoglobin (Hb) A1c levels measured within the past 6 months, or low-density lipoprotein (LDL)-cholesterol levels measured in the past 12 months. Physicians in the control group had access to usual clinical education relating to the care of patients with diabetes. At baseline, no significant differences were found in HbA1c levels, LDL-cholesterol levels or blood-pressure levels, or with adherence to HbA1c- or LDL-cholesterol-monitoring guidelines between patients. At completion of the study, patients cared for by physicians in the intervention group were more likely to have had HbA1c levels measured within 6 months (61.5% versus 48.1%), and more likely to have had LDL-cholesterol levels measured within 12 months (75.8% versus 64.1%), compared with patients cared for by physicians in the control group. HbA1c, LDL-cholesterol and blood-pressure levels were similar in patients cared for by physicians in the two groups. The findings of the study demonstrated how registry-based audit, feedback and patient reminders can improve adherence to treatment recommendations for diabetes care.

8.5 Conclusion

This chapter described the characteristics of five forms of evaluation: proactive, clarificative, interactive, monitoring, and impact. These provide a conceptual map for evaluators, providers, consumers and other relevant individuals about how to proceed with an evaluation activity. While it is possible to evaluate all stages of a program cycle, from design and development to implementation, it is more common to select one specific form. The type of decision made depends on the kinds of questions that need to be asked about the program and the concerns of the consumers and other stakeholders.

8.6 DISCUSSION QUESTIONS

1. Define the following terms: goal, outcome, strategy, objective, performance indicator, and performance measure.
2. Differentiate between the following forms of evaluation in terms of purpose, timing and approaches used: proactive, clarificative, interactive, monitoring, and impact evaluation.
3. Hospital Y has been running a nurse-led cardiac clinic for 3 years. The hospital managers wish to determine how adequately the clinic has served patients' needs and the extent to which anticipated goals have been met. Describe how an evaluation could be undertaken to address the managers' concerns.
4. University lecturers have identified that their Bachelor of Nursing curriculum is too content-laden and teacher-centred. They decide to change it to a problem-based learning approach, with the focus on student-centred needs. The lecturers wish to determine how to use the characteristics of problem-based learning in developing their new curriculum. Describe how an evaluation could be undertaken in this situation.

8.7 References

Brandon P R 1999 Involving program stakeholders in reviews of evaluators' recommendations for program revisions. *Evaluation and Program Planning* 22(3):363–72.

Bucknall T, Manias E, Botti M 2001 Acute pain management: the implications of scientific evidence for nursing practice in the postoperative context. *International Journal of Nursing Practice* 7(4):266–73.

Centers for Disease Control and Prevention 1999 Framework for program evaluation in public health. *Morbidity and Mortality Weekly Report* 48(RR–11, September):17.

Colton D 1997 The design of evaluations for continuous quality improvement. *Evaluation and the Health Professions* 20(3):265–85.

Department of Health and Aged Care 2001 *Evaluation: a guide for good practice.* Commonwealth of Australia, Canberra.

Dickinson A, Welch C, Ager L 2008 No longer hungry in hospital: improving the hospital mealtime experience for older people through action research. *Journal of Clinical Nursing* 17(11):1492–502.

Dornan T, Arno M, Hadfield J et al 2006 Student evaluation of the clinical 'curriculum in action'. *Medical Educator* 40(7):667–74.

Elixhauser A, Halpern M, Schmier J et al 1998 Health care CBA and CEA from 1991 to 1996: an updated bibliography. *Medical Care* 36(suppl 5):MS1–9.

Ellis R, Hogard E 2003 Two deficits and a solution? Explicating and evaluating clinical facilitation using consultative methods and multiple stakeholder perspectives. *Learning in Health and Social Care* 2(1):18–27.

Fleming M L, Parker E 2007 *Health promotion: principles and practice in the Australian context, 3rd edn.* Allen & Unwin, Sydney.

Green L W 1990 *Community health,* 6th edn. Times Mirror/CV Mosby College, St Louis.

Greenwood D J, Levin M 2006 *Introduction to action research: social research for social change, 2nd edn.* Sage Publications, London.

Grembowski D 2001 *The practice of health program evaluation.* Sage Publications, Thousand Oaks, CA.

Guba E, Lincoln Y 1981 *Effective evaluation.* Jossey-Bass, San Francisco, CA.

Guba E, Lincoln Y 1989 *Fourth generation evaluation.* Sage Publications, London.

Hulscher M, Wensing M, Grol R et al 1999 Interventions to improve the delivery of preventative services in primary care. *American Journal of Public Health* 89(5):737–46.

Joint Commission on Accreditation of Healthcare Organizations & National Pharmaceutical Council 2003 *Improving the quality of pain management through measurement and action.* Joint Commission on Accreditation of Healthcare Organizations, Oakbrook Terrace, IL.

Manias E, Aitken R 2003 Achieving collaborative workplace learning in a university critical care course. *Intensive and Critical Care Nursing* 19(1):50–61.

Manias E, Aitken R, Dunning T 2005 How graduate nurses use protocols to manage patients' medications. *Journal of Clinical Nursing* 14(8):935–44.

Manias E, Bullock S 2002 The educational preparation of undergraduate nursing students in pharmacology: clinical nurses' perceptions and experiences of graduate nurses' medication knowledge. *International Journal of Nursing Studies* 39(8):773–84.

Manias E, Bullock S, Bennett R 2000 Formative evaluation of a computer assisted learning program in pharmacology for nursing students. *Computers in Nursing* 18(6):265–71.

Owen J M 2006 *Program evaluation: forms and approaches, 3rd edn.* Allen & Unwin, Sydney.

Owen J M, Rogers P J 1999 *Program evaluation: forms and approaches, international edn.* Sage Publications, London.

Patton M Q 2002 *Qualitative research and evaluation methods, 3rd edn.* Sage Publications, Beverly Hills, CA.

Reason, P, Bradbury, H (eds) 2007 *The Sage handbook of action research: participatory inquiry and practice.* Sage Publications, London.

Reid R J 2000 A cost–benefit analysis of syringe exchange programs. *Journal of Health & Social Policy* 11(4):41–57.

Rice T H 2007 Measuring health care costs and trends. In: R M Anderson, T H Rice, G F Kominski (eds) *Changing the US health care system: key issues in health services, policy and management, 3rd edn.* Jossey-Bass, San Francisco, CA, pp. 117–34.

Roth J 1990 Needs and the needs assessment process. *Evaluation Practice* 11(2):39–44.

Scheirer M A 1998 Commentary: evaluation planning is the heart of the matter. *The American Journal of Evaluation* 19(3):385–91.

Thomas K G, Thomas M R, Stroebel R J et al 2007 Use of registry-generated audit, feedback, and patient reminder intervention in an internal medicine resident clinic – a randomised controlled trial. *Journal of General Internal Medicine* 22(12):1740–4.

Thorogood M, Coombes Y 2006 *Evaluating health promotion: practice and methods, 2nd edn.* Oxford University Press, Oxford.

Wadsworth Y 1997 *Everyday evaluation on the run, 2nd edn.* Allen & Unwin, Sydney.

PART FIVE

Translating evidence into practice

CHAPTER 9

Evidence to inform nursing practice: An applied approach

Colleen Smith, Kate Andre, Kelly Lewis and Barbara Parker

9.1 Learning objectives

After reading this chapter, you should be able to:

1. understand the health professional's role in ensuring that a care pathway is based on the most contemporary, up-to-date knowledge and is contextual to the client group and available resources
2. understand the critical reflective process and its application in the utilisation of evidence-based practice (EBP), and
3. demonstrate how the evidence-based process can be applied to review a care pathway.

9.2 Introduction

The use of evidence to inform nursing practice and improve patient outcomes is gaining momentum. The benefits of this approach are realised, as increasing numbers of students and clinicians are exposed to evidence-based practice (EBP) in their education and practice areas. As a result, clinical decision making is now more likely to be based on information derived from research. Care pathways are one example of a clinical tool that, when developed from the best available evidence, can improve clinical effectiveness and efficiency.

The purpose of this chapter is to showcase an approach that clinicians and students may use to obtain evidence to justify the need for a more extensive EBP process. After setting the scene through a discussion of clinical pathways, the authors situate the EBP approach within a framework of critical reflection guided by a series of reflective questions. Next, a case study is used to highlight how the approach can be used to examine a clinical question arising from practice. The case study uses a component of a care pathway for a client presenting for an elective total hip replacement. The chapter concludes with a scenario-based activity that can be used to apply what has been learned.

9.3 Care pathways and evidence for nursing practice

Within the context of the clinical setting, evidence-based nursing refers to the identification of specific nursing practices that may require further development, and the accessing and evaluation of current evidence to make recommendations for improvement (Courtney 2005). Regardless of the approach used to initiate changes in practice, all aspects of patient care, where possible, should be based upon the best available evidence. The following section will provide an overview of how care pathways are useful in supporting and assisting health professionals in using current EBP.

9.3.1 Using care pathways to inform quality nursing practice

The terms clinical pathways, critical pathways, care maps and integrated care pathways are often used interchangeably to describe health management plans that assimilate information from a variety of sources (Panella et al 2003). These pathways provide a step-by-step guide for health professionals to work through both contextual and practical issues of client care (Whittle & Hewison 2007). A pathway should be designed using current evidence to identify and evaluate goals of care, and provide the sequence and timing of nursing interventions required to achieve the best possible health outcomes for the patient (Middleton et al 2001). The use of care pathways allows health professionals to improve patient health outcomes by ensuring that no aspect of care is overlooked. In addition, care pathways provide a baseline record against which improvement or deterioration may be judged, and move the patient towards discharge in a timely and consistent manner. Variations in expected outcomes of care are documented and these data are essential in monitoring and preventing adverse outcomes or delays in discharge. In turn, this assists healthcare professionals in ensuring that they are following safe practice guidelines. The step-by-step approach of care pathways enables nursing staff to work through prescriptive guidelines for assessment, planning and evaluation of patient progress specific to the patient's condition (Campbell et al 1998, Panella et al 2003). Emphasis is placed on the provision of appropriate care in relation to the clinical evidence base, clinical guidelines and/or consensus of best practice. In this way, care pathways provide standards that help reduce unnecessary variations in patient care and outcomes (Middleton et al 2001).

Evaluation of care pathways has demonstrated that the use of this approach can significantly improve the quality of many clinical processes, both directly and indirectly (Panella et al 2003). Patients who are cared for using a care pathway report greater satisfaction with their care and receive more information and education about their condition (Whittle & Hewison 2007). In addition to this, care pathways have been shown to encourage review of current practice and adoption of most recent evidence to improve patient care (Campbell et al 1998, Panella et al 2003). Review of pathway documentation and medical records for common surgical procedures reveals that much of the benefit of using this type of approach comes from the development stage and not necessarily from sustained utilisation. As such, this development and review activity is clearly important because it can be the stimulus to promote communication between health professionals and implementation of best practice (Dy et al 2005).

9.3.2 Care pathways and the application of evidence to practice

As stated above, care pathways have been systematically developed to assist healthcare professionals in making decisions, based on summaries of the best available evidence (Middleton et al 2001, Whittle & Hewison 2007). They assist in the provision of quality care through providing a foundation and framework for decision making, thus reducing variation in clinical practice (Middleton et al 2001, Miller & Kearney 2004). However, it is important to be aware that care pathways, like other clinical practice guidelines, have limitations, and that those not based on solid up-to-date evidence may significantly impact on the quality of patient outcomes (Middleton et al 2001, Miller & Kearney 2004). Clinicians who care for patients must be informed on current standards of practice, because it is their role as a healthcare professional to assess the quality of evidence on which interventions are based (Courtney 2005). The process of appraising current practice-based interventions, determining their validity and applicability, and placing this information within the context of patient need, will provide a solid foundation for the development of lifelong learning skills and future improvements in patient care outcomes (Courtney 2005, Sanderlin & AbdulRahim 2007). Critical reflection is a useful strategy to assist this process as it requires clinicians to question their practice in order to expose underlying assumptions and the taken-for-granted aspects of their work. Through a questioning attitude combined with an EBP approach, new knowledge emerges to inform practice change.

9.4 Reflection and evidence-based practice

Critical reflection and EBP are important elements for professional practice. Embedding the critical reflective process into EBP provides the foundation and framework for decision making in clinical practice (Barredo 2005). Care pathways are one of many tools available for use in the clinical practice setting (Courtney 2005). All clinical tools should be developed and appraised using a rigorous stepwise process (Courtney 2005).

9.4.1 Knowledge and experience

When you set out to evaluate a clinical tool, such as a care pathway, you will need to engage in the process of reflective questioning to establish what you already know about EBP and the topic you are investigating. You may wish to consider the following questions when undertaking this process:

- Do I understand the relationship between research, knowledge and professional practice?
- What knowledge do I need to safely and comprehensively care for the patient described in the care pathway?
- If I identify that I have gaps in my knowledge base and/or experience, how do I address this?
- How can I access, evaluate and incorporate literature to increase my knowledge and understanding?
- What does this mean for my professional practice?

9.4.2 Care pathway model

Patient groups who suit the care pathway model are those patients who follow a predictable course (Middleton et al 2001). Therefore, you will need to determine if the care pathway is an accurate reflection of your patient's needs (Every et al 2000). You will also need to consider how strong the evidence is that has been used to develop and create the care pathway (Every et al 2000, Middleton et al 2001, Sanderlin & AbdulRahim 2007). When applying the theory of EBP for the evaluation of a clinical tool, such as a care pathway, further questions you may ask are:

- What is the purpose of the care pathway?
- Who is the target group?
- Is the pathway an accurate reflection of patient need?

- How do I know the pathway is up to date (i.e. is it likely to account for important recent developments)?
- How do I know if the evidence is both current and correctly applied?
- How strong is the quality of evidence used in the development of the pathway?
- Is the pathway an accurate reflection of the appraised evidence?
- Has the pathway been subjected to peer review?
- Do I know how often a care pathway should be reviewed?
- When was the pathway previously reviewed?
- Where can I find this information (Courtney 2005, Every et al 2000, Middleton et al 2001, Middleton & Roberts 2000)?

This questioning technique highlights what you need to know in order to develop a new care pathway and/or evaluate an existing one. It also informs decisions about the appropriateness of the pathway within the context of patient need. Furthermore, it exposes the strengths and deficits in your own knowledge and practice.

9.4.3 Evidence-based decision making

Decision making involves deciding upon an action after considering the risks and benefits of the various alternatives (Thompson et al 2004). Evidence-based decision making incorporates alternatives and, hence, the associated risks and benefits, from a combination of clinical knowledge and expertise, patient preference, evidence, and available resources (DiCenso et al 1998). Developing clinical questions is the first step in the EBP process (Stone 2002). Having evaluated the key questions described above, you will need to establish whether you have enough evidence and knowledge to safely and comprehensively care for the patient (Craig et al 2001). At this point, it is important to consider the purpose of the pathway review, as well as the type of evidence you require to evaluate and critique the relevance of the care pathway and determine its appropriateness for use in a particular clinical situation.

Investigating the purpose of the pathway review is important (Every et al 2000), because this will influence the extent of your literature search and review, as well as the extent to which this information may be applied to the practice/policy of the institution. If you are submitting a report to your 'care pathways development committee' and undertaking a systematic review, for example, then the purpose of this activity is to provide an exhaustive review of all the relevant literature in order to inform a change at an institutional level. If this is the case, you would need to use a range of search engines to retrieve and review all the relevant literature, as outlined in Chapter 6. Depending on the number of relevant research publications, this can be a very time-consuming process. Alternatively, as in the case study that follows, if the purpose is an initial examination of evidence in response to a clinical question—and possibly to advise those responsible for the review/development of care pathways, as a consequence of the information you find—the extent of your review may be limited. Assuming that this is the situation and the time you have to commit to the situation is not extensive, it would be appropriate to review the literature and retrieve three or four highly related research articles with a strong evidence base to review. It is not feasible to always undertake an exhaustive search and review of the literature given the time constraints inherent in clinical practice; however, it is important that the extent of the literature review is reflected in how the evidence retrieved is applied to practice. For instance, in the case study that follows, it is only feasible to undertake a limited search and retrieve the most accessible of articles (as opposed to an exhaustive search and retrieval of the literature). As a consequence, the application of the information provided needs to reflect this. For example, the advice you will give the client should be framed as, 'Based on the four articles I have read on the subject, there is evidence that …..' If you identify the need to extend or adjust the care pathway, then it is appropriate you inform those responsible for care pathway development so they can conduct a more extensive review and attend to a potential deficit.

In considering the type of evidence and its appropriateness to a clinical situation, you may wish to consider the following questions:

- What characteristics of your patient are important (i.e. diagnosis, patient preference, procedures, age, prior illness)?
- What interventions are you interested in?
- What alternatives do you want to compare your intervention to?
- What measurable outcomes are you interested in (Craig et al 2001)?

In order to evaluate the appropriateness of the existing evidence and answer the specific questions you have developed, you require accurate and reliable information (Courtney 2005, Craig et al 2001, Middleton et al 2001, Middleton & Roberts 2000). Therefore, the next step in this process is to consider how you will find the best type of available and relevant evidence to achieve this (Miller & Kearney 2004). When searching for evidence to evaluate the efficacy of a care pathway, you will need to consider implementing a systematic process to enable the location and identification of the required information (Courtney 2005, Craig et al 2001, Middleton et al 2001, Middleton & Roberts 2000). The following questions should assist you with this:

- Is there any research available that could be used?
- What type of primary research data will you access?
- What is the quality of the research evidence available?
- Has the research been incorporated into a systematic review? Is the highest level of evidence available?
- What type of evidence-based information might you access from your clinical setting or other clinical settings/health institutions?
- If you are unable to locate primary research data, what other information might you consider?
- Where might you look for this (Courtney 2005, Craig et al 2001)?

After you have completed your search for evidence, the strengths and weaknesses of the research must be evaluated (Courtney 2005, Miller & Kearney 2004). Critically appraising the quality of the material found is an extremely important step in the EBP process as it facilitates decision making regarding the incorporation of new information into clinical practice (Craig et al 2001, Miller & Kearney 2004). This will assist you in determining whether the information located is valid and useful to enhance the quality of care in the clinical setting (Miller & Kearney 2004). This process will also assist you to compare the evidence with current management and existing practice, and determine the appropriateness of the care pathway content. To complete this process, you will need to consider the rigorous strategies required to critically appraise evidence and then synthesise this information, developing a summary of the existing knowledge (Courtney 2005, Craig et al 2001).

Figure 9.1 is an example of a component of a care pathway you may encounter for a client undergoing total hip replacement surgery, in particular, the preoperative assessment. You can see how important it is that current evidence is employed to determine these interventions and outcomes, as this tool guides staff in the total care required for these clients. Variations to the expected outcomes need to be identified and documented, and in some cases information is provided in the care pathway regarding how to manage these events.

Diagnosis: Total hip replacement	UR:		WARD:
DATE: _____	SURNAME:		OTHER NAMES:
Pre-operative assessment component ONLY	DOB:	SEX:	MEDICAL OFFICER:

CARE CATEGORIES	INTERVENTION AND OUTCOME STATEMENTS	Initial where outcome is met. Provide details where not met.
Consults	Anaesthetist review complete Surgical team review complete	
Investigations	Pre-operative CBE LFTs and other blood samples taken Autologous blood collection booked X-rays reviewed and additional images undertaken 12-lead ECG completed and submitted to anaesthetist to review MSSU: equipment and instruction provided – to be completed 2 weeks prior to surgery and managed by GP – if necessary antibiotic course completed prior to admission Patient measured for below-knee TED stockings	
Observations	Vital signs and oxygen saturation taken/recorded on preoperative assessment sheet and in normal limits	
Psycho/Social and discharge plan	Patient/family education complete including: • surgical procedure and likely postoperative experience • admission procedure night before surgery • discharge possibilities (home with support or rehabilitative facility)	
Medications	Patient provided with information sheet including: • warfarin/aspirin/NSAID to cease 5–7 days preoperative or as directed by surgeon/anaesthetist (details written on sheet) • all other prescribed medications to continue as per medical orders	
Risk assessment	Risk assessment sheet complete Smoking cessation plan provided where appropriate	

Figure 9.1 Care pathway: Preoperative assessment component for elective total hip replacement

9.5 Application to practice

Using the case study detailed as follows, this section will take you through the applied process of developing a clinical question, and how this in turn informs the search for evidence.

CASE STUDY

You are a recently qualified registered nurse working in a preoperative assessment clinic, reading the case record of Mrs Martin aged 75 years who has an afternoon appointment. The record reveals that Mrs Martin lives alone in a house she has occupied for the past 50 years. She has a history of right hip pain that radiates down her leg, resulting in reduced mobility. Over the past few months, the intensity of the pain has increased, making it more difficult for her to mobilise. She is moderately overweight and was diagnosed with severe degenerative arthritis of the right hip 2 years ago. Her daughter, who works full time, lives in a nearby suburb and visits her on the weekends and takes her for a drive.

Since the death of her husband 6 years ago, Mrs Martin has been suffering moderate depression, which has been treated by her local general practitioner. Her medication regimen includes a non-steroidal anti-inflammatory drug (NSAID) for her arthritic pain and an antidepressant drug. Last week she was seen by an orthopaedic surgeon who recommended she have a total hip replacement. Mrs Martin agreed to the surgery and it has been scheduled for 8 weeks' time. An appointment has been made for her to attend a pre-admission clinic for preoperative assessment.

You access the clinical pathway for elective total hip replacement and notice that the preoperative assessment component of the pathway (see Fig 9.1) does not include an exercise program as part of preoperative patient education. As a nursing student, you recall a conversation you had with a physiotherapist (while on an orthopaedic ward placement) who pointed out that patients who undertook an exercise program prior to undergoing hip replacement surgery had stronger upper and lower body muscles and mobilised more quickly postoperatively, leading to earlier discharge. You discuss this with the clinic manager, who is supportive of further discussion and investigation of the influence of preoperative exercise programs. You volunteer to search for evidence and refer back to a textbook you used last year when you did a course on EBP in your undergraduate degree. The textbook describes a series of steps to guide the process and includes:

- developing a clinical question
- locating the evidence
- critically appraising the evidence
- implementing evidence in practice, and
- evaluating patient outcomes and the process.

9.5.1 Developing a clinical question

While reading about the development of a clinical question, you note that a vital part of EBP involves spending time developing an appropriate and relevant clinical question to yield the best available evidence. You know that if your question is too ambiguous you will have difficulty in locating the evidence, which may lead to irrelevant information. A clear, concise question will make it easier for you to generate the best available evidence and avoid wasting time.

The PICO method (described in Ch 5) is one format you can use to develop clinical questions. You like this format because it is similar to the one you used during your studies to develop a research question for a research simulation group work project. The PICO method has four parts:

- P: Patient, population or problem
- I: Intervention or independent variables
- C: Comparison
- O: Outcomes (Stone 2002).

Your first attempt produces the following clinical question:

> Do 75-year-old clients having a total hip replacement (P) who exercise before surgery (I) go home earlier (O) compared with those who don't exercise (C)?

You discuss the question with your clinical manager, who raises the following questions:

- What do you mean by exercise; for example, do you mean aerobic exercise or strength-training exercise?
- Is there any reason why clients less than 75 years old would be different to those older than 75 years? Why do you need to limit your search to this age group?
- Is it feasible that those having an emergency total hip replacement would choose to undertake an exercise program prior to surgery?
- While the outcome may be that the client goes home earlier, is this really the specific client outcome that you are looking for?
- What surgical procedure are your comparative client group undergoing?
- What search terms will you use to locate the literature?

9.5.2 Locating the evidence

You appreciate the discussion and feedback, and a further attempt produces a refined question comprising each part of the PICO method with measurable and observable components. The refined question becomes:

> **1. Research question**
> For older adult patients undergoing elective surgery for total hip replacement (P), does the performance of a muscle-strengthening exercise program preoperatively (I) reduce the time taken to mobilise without nursing assistance in the postoperative period (O) compared with total hip replacement patients who have not undertaken an exercise program (C)?

Your question has pertinence for nurses and other medical and allied health professionals, so you decide to conduct a search of the Cochrane, CINAHL® and MEDLINE® databases. You proceed to plan a search strategy by extracting keywords from the clinical question that include the problem and the intervention.

> **2. Extracting keywords**
> | | |
> |---|---|
> | Cochrane Database of Systematic Reviews | arthroplasty hip |
> | | exercise |
> | CINAHL | arthroplasty |
> | | exercise |
> | MEDLINE | arthroplasty |
> | | exercise |

You enter these keywords using the 'Advanced Search' option in each database. You also use the following limiters specific to each database:

3. Limiting the search	
Cochrane Database of Systematic Reviews	You combine your keywords with the Boolean operator **AND**
CINAHL	Apply related words ✓ Publication year: **(from 2000–2008)** Peer reviewed ✓ Research article ✓ Age groups: **(Aged, 65+ years)** This search brings up a list of related major subject headings. You select the term **'Arthroplasty, Replacement, Hip'** to further refine the search.
MEDLINE	You search each keyword separately in the following way: Keyword: **arthroplasty** Map term to subject heading ✓ This search brings up a list of related major subject headings. You tick the term **'Arthroplasty, Replacement, Hip'** and choose 'explode' to further refine the search. You further limit the search to: Humans: ✓ Publication year: **(2000–2008)** Age groups: **All aged (65 and over)** You now start a new search for your next keyword: Keyword: **exercise** Map term to subject heading ✓ This search brings up a list of related major subject headings. You tick the term **'Exercise therapy'** and choose 'explode' to further refine the search. You further limit the search to: Humans: ✓ Publication year: **(2000–2008)** Age groups: **All aged (65 and over)** You are now ready to combine the two separate keyword searches. Opening the search history reveals four separate searches. You tick the following two searches and select 'combine': Search #2 Arthroplasty/or exp Arthroplasty, Replacement, Hip, limit 1 to humans and yr = "2000–2008" and All aged (65 and over) Search #4 Exercise/or exp Exercise Therapy, limit 3 to humans and yr = "2000–2008" and All aged (65 and over)

Database	Search 1	Search 2
Cochrane Database of Systematic Reviews (Cochrane Reviews)	25	0
CINAHL	27	11
MEDLINE	34	5

Table 9.1 Search strategy results

Your first search retrieves the results indicated in Table 9.1 and you note there are a large number of articles. Looking at the results, you question if some of these results could appear in more than one database, accounting for the large numbers. If you search several databases it is possible that you will retrieve some of the same publications, so you check this and further limit the number of articles. To limit your search even further, you add more keywords to the original search that describe the clinical question outcome measure (you enter the keywords 'mobility' and 'function'), obtaining a smaller number of articles.

With a quick review of the article abstracts with reference to the clinical question and hierarchy of evidence, you further limit to the most relevant studies. There are no systematic reviews so you proceed to retrieve the full-text version of randomised controlled trials (RCTs), which you decided were the best form of evidence to answer the clinical question.

---

4. Retrieve the full-text version of the selected articles

Cochrane Database of Systematic Reviews (Cochrane Reviews)	RCTs in Cochrane can be retrieved simply by clicking on 'Record'.
CINAHL	Use the pdf icon if available to open the full text. Refer to Chapter 5 (Section 5.5.6) for other options.
MEDLINE	Use the link to the full text on the right-hand side of your search results.

The articles you retrieve from the systematic search strategy outlined above are:
1. Gilbey H J, Ackland T R, Wang A W et al 2003 Exercise improves early functional recovery after total hip arthroplasty. *Clinical Orthopaedics & Related Research* 408:193–200.
2. Rooks D S, Huang J, Bierbaum B E et al 2006 Effect of preoperative exercise on measures of functional status in men and women undergoing total hip and knee arthroplasty. *Arthritis & Rheumatism: Arthritis Care & Research* 55(5):700–8.
3. Wang A W, Gilbey H J, Ackland T R 2002 Perioperative exercise programs improve early return of ambulatory function after total hip arthroplasty: a randomized, controlled trial. *American Journal of Physical Medicine & Rehabilitation* 81(11):801–6.
4. Whitney J A, Parkman S 2002 Preoperative physical activity, anesthesia, and analgesia: effects on early postoperative walking after total hip replacement. *Applied Nursing Research* 15(1):19–27.

9.5.3 Critically appraising the evidence

You read that critical appraisal is an integral part of determining the quality of research evidence and that various tools have been established to assist researchers and healthcare professionals in this process (Courtney 2005). These tools may be applied to quantitative and qualitative research studies, systematic reviews and clinical guidelines (Courtney 2005). From your reading, you are also reminded of the importance of selecting the appropriate appraisal tool for the method of the study under investigation, so that the evidence gained from this process can be used as a benchmark to inform practice (Courtney 2005).

You choose the four articles noted above for critical appraisal because of their relevance in addressing your research question. In particular, each article details empirical research specific to the effects of preoperative exercise followed by hip arthroplasty. The nature of the question—namely, the physical benefits of a preoperative exercise program on postoperative functional recovery—dictates your decision to evaluate empirical research. If the question had required inclusion of the patient's perceptions of the experience of the exercise program (e.g. why patients chose to participate in a program) then you would have chosen to appraise qualitative studies.

You use the Critical Appraisal Skills Program (CASP) tool (see www.phru.nhs.uk /Pages/PHD/resources.htm) to review the four RCTs. You select the CASP because it provides a clear and systematic approach for examining the studies. This tool utilises ten broad questions to guide the appraisal process. The first two questions are screening questions that allow you to decide if you will proceed with the remaining eight questions. The questions are as follows:

1. Did the study ask a clearly-focused question? (screening question)
2. Was this an RCT and was it appropriately so? (screening question)
3. Were participants appropriately allocated to intervention and control groups?
4. Were participants, staff and study personnel 'blind' to participants' study groups?
5. Were all of the participants who entered the trial accounted for at its conclusion?
6. Were the participants in all groups followed up and data collected in the same way?
7. Did the study have enough participants to minimise the play of chance?
8. How are the results presented and what is the main result?
9. How precise are these results?
10. Were all important outcomes considered so the results can be applied?

As you undertake each critical appraisal, you compile a summary of the study, the findings and your appraisal so that you can consider decisions regarding the implementation of the evidence into practice. The following is your summary of the appraised evidence.

9.5.3.1 Study 1

The article by Gilbey et al (2003) used a prospective randomised design to determine if a structured pre- and post-surgery exercise program for total hip arthroplasty patients improved muscular strength and early functional recovery compared with a control group who received no additional exercise apart from the routine in-hospital physical therapy. The sample initially comprised 76 patients with end-stage hip arthritis. Excluded were patients with a history of hip infection, a significant neuromuscular disease, hip malignancy, poor general health and those who required revised hip surgery and bilateral hip replacement. The final sample comprised 57 patients: 32 in the intervention group and 25 in the control group.

All patients underwent a baseline assessment in week 8 prior to surgery and there was no significant difference between the intervention and control groups. Patients in the intervention group did two supervised and two unsupervised exercise sessions per week for 8 weeks prior to surgery. The two supervised sessions recommenced 3 weeks post-surgery and patients were encouraged to continue the two unsupervised sessions. Various instruments were used to measure the outcomes, which included muscle strength, hip flexion range of motion and physical function. Gilbey et al (2003) concluded that an exercise program commencing 8 weeks prior to surgery improved each of the three outcome measures. The continuation of the exercise program post-surgery maintained this functional advantage for up to 6 months when compared with patients who received the routine pre- and post-surgery care.

Applying the CASP appraisal tool highlighted there was no blinding of patient group allocation for clinicians who performed the pre- and postoperative assessment. According to Courtney (2005), this can introduce data collector bias for the outcome measured. The findings are limited to patients who are motivated and able to attend the clinic and partake in the exercise program. There was no indication as to how the randomisation process was done, nor was there any mention of the reliability and validity of the instruments used.

9.5.3.2 Study 2

The study conducted by Rooks et al (2006) used a similar design to determine the effectiveness of a 6-week preoperative exercise program on the level of pre- and postoperative function, pain and muscle strength. Of a possible 942 patients who met the inclusion criteria, 108 men and women undergoing total hip arthroplasty or total knee arthroplasty were randomised to one of two treatment groups. The intervention group participated in a total body fitness program of cardiovascular, strength and flexibility training, three times a week for the 6 weeks immediately prior to the surgical procedure. The control group was provided with education including written information on how to reduce the risk of postoperative falls and injury, and one follow-up telephone call.

The results clearly show a benefit from undertaking an exercise regimen preoperatively for subjects undergoing a total hip arthroplasty. Exercise participation increased muscle strength preoperatively, whereas the control patients recorded no perceptible change in strength. In addition, undertaking the exercise routine prior to total joint arthroplasty was shown to increase the likelihood of discharge home and reduce the incidence of discharge to a rehabilitation facility.

Again, applying the CASP tool, it was possible to determine the strengths and limitations of this study. The strengths of the study were that it was a randomised, controlled design. Blinding of testers to patient group assignment was ensured and standardised tools used to assess outcome measures. The use of a single site contributed to the consistency of treatment implementation and data collection. The limitations included a low recruitment rate (12%) for the number of eligible patients and a high attrition rate (28%); however, the authors accounted for all withdrawals. In addition, the study design may prejudice those subjects unable to fulfil some requirements of the study (e.g. travel), because subjects who are usually sedentary, and have previously been found to show larger gains from exercise, were not highly represented in the sample. The ability to capture this group may have affected the outcomes of this study and decreased the generalisability of the results.

9.5.3.3 Study 3

The study by Wang et al (2002) again was a prospective randomised design where subjects were allocated to either an 'exercise' or 'routine care' group post-total hip arthroplasty. The exercise program commenced 8 weeks prior to the surgery and included two supervised clinic-based classes and two home-based exercise sessions each week. The sample size was 28, with 15 allocated to the intervention group and 13 to the control. Exclusion criteria and measurement activities were as per Gilbey et al (2003). These two studies have very similar foundations.

The results of the study indicated that those who had undertaken the scheduled exercise program demonstrated greater ambulatory function that was potentially sufficient to enhance the rate of recovery and possibly discharge. The CASP appraisal process highlighted the same outcomes as per Gilbey et al (2003). The subjects within this study shared considerable similarities to those associated with the question (e.g. same age profile, elective total hip replacement as a consequence of arthritic conditions).

9.5.3.4 Study 4

The final article chosen, Whitney and Parkman (2002), was similarly selected because of its empirical study design and relevance to the topic. This RCT was designed to investigate whether self-reported preoperative physical activity, type of anaesthesia (epidural, general or combination) and postoperative analgesia (continuous epidural or patient-controlled morphine) influenced distances walked in the first 3 days after total hip arthroscopy. The central focus of the study was a postoperative intervention to improve walking distances and, as such, the preoperative exercise routines (self-reported) were subject to a secondary analysis separate from the randomised design.

The sample included 58 subjects aged 45–79 years who underwent a total hip arthroplasty for the treatment of osteoarthritis. Subjects were randomly assigned postoperatively to either a standard exercise program (control) or 4 days of augmented physical activity postoperatively (intervention). For those subjects assigned to the intervention group, the physical activity program included isometric exercises for the gluteus, quadriceps, biceps and triceps muscles, designed to enhance walking capabilities postoperatively. All subjects followed a walking protocol, increasing distance on a daily basis. Distances walked were reported via the physical therapy progress reports within the medical notes and a bedside activity diary kept by the primary nurse and investigative team members (seen twice daily).

The results revealed that 63% of the control group and 71% of the intervention group reported to be inactive preoperatively; this is higher than the sedentary rate for the general population (40%), possibly due in part to the pain of their condition. In both the control and intervention groups, those subjects who reported higher activity levels before surgery were able to walk greater distances postoperatively. Importantly, there was a correlation between longer distances walked postoperatively and shorter hospital stays. There was, however, no identified link between the types of anaesthesia or postoperative pain relief received and postoperative mobility.

Again, applying the CASP tool, it was possible to determine the strengths and limitations of this study. Although this was a randomised, controlled design, it is important to note that the data relevant to the clinical question you have posed; namely, the self-reporting of preoperative exercise, was not part of this design. However, if the clinical question was about encouraging patients to undertake a general exercise program preoperatively, this aspect of the study may be relevant. Self-reporting of health-related behaviours is potentially unreliable; however, this does not completely invalidate these findings. Nevertheless, it is important to note that this study was not able to adjust for the impact of the subjects' underlying condition on their preoperative exercise tolerance, and the potential bias that those with greater levels of incapacity (and hence less likely to exercise preoperatively) were also likely to have reduced postoperative recovery for reasons unrelated to their preoperative exercise. In other words, it is not possible to say from this study that preoperative exercise was an independent factor in determining a patient's ability to walk greater distances postoperatively. It is clear, however, that a patient who is in better health preoperatively, and hence more likely to be active, is also likely to be in better health postoperatively.

The review of the four articles using the CASP tool allows you to consider your clinical question in light of the evidence. From the information collected in the articles, you can see that there is some evidence that in older adult clients undergoing a total hip arthroplasty (P) the performance of a muscle-strengthening exercise program preoperatively (I) may reduce the time taken to mobilise without nursing assistance in the postoperative period (O) compared with clients who have not undertaken an exercise program (C). In particular, a structured 6–8-week exercise program described by Gilbey et al (2003), Rooks et al (2006) and Wang (2002) was shown to have benefits on postoperative mobilisation. Whitney and Parkman (2002) did not clearly demonstrate that having patients increase their exercise preoperatively was plausible, nor did they demonstrate that preoperative exercise (separate from other comorbidities, for example) was an independent predictor of improvements of postoperative walking. However, they did demonstrate a correlation between an increase in walking distance postoperatively and shortened hospital stay (Whitney & Parkman 2002), which has some relevance to the clinical question you asked. None of these studies assessed the time taken to mobilise without nursing assistance, and therefore have limited relevance to the question posed.

9.5.4 Implementing evidence in practice and evaluating the process and patient outcomes

Now that you have used the evidence-based nursing practice approach to critique a care pathway and determine the currency, applicability and appropriateness of the information that you have found, you will need to consider how the evidence you have discovered can be implemented into practice. You decide that the level of evidence is sufficient for you to bring your findings to the attention of those responsible for the implementation of structural change at the organisational level. This group could then undertake a more extensive investigation involving a systematic review in order to inform decisions about the inclusion of a preoperative exercise program as part of the clinical pathway. It is beyond the scope of this chapter to elaborate on the process your organisation would need to implement change in clinical practice at this level; however, it is clear that the registered nurse at the grass roots level can be an important catalyst for stimulating this change.

In summary, it is important that all health professionals access and utilise evidence to extend and support their practice. However, it is not feasible in situations where a systematic review is not available (e.g. through the Joanna Briggs Institute) for clinical staff to expend copious hours in this activity. Rather, there are situations that call for a sound and appropriate search of the literature, where a range of quality articles are accessed and used to inform a local issue or initiate a more extensive review. This case study represents such an approach. The outcome of a review where four appropriate articles have been sourced and evaluated can be the stimulus for an organisation to consider providing the resources to fully investigate the evidence. Therefore, don't be reticent about providing the outcome of your review process to those responsible for instigating this within your organisation.

9.6 Conclusion

Within the context of the clinical setting, evidence-based nursing refers to the identification of specific nursing practices that may require further development, and the accessing and evaluation of current evidence to make recommendations for improvement. Care pathways may be a useful tool to guide health professionals in implementing evidence-based treatment for specific client groups. In this chapter, we have described the importance of the combination of critical thinking skills and experience required by nurses to determine appropriate care for any client. In so doing, we have presented a step-by-step process to assist novice nurses to access, apply and evaluate information to ensure that nursing care is based on the most contemporary, up-to-date knowledge and is contextual to the client group and available resources. Variations exist in client care and this process must allow for nurses to critique the best available evidence in light of individual clinical expertise and patient preferences. The application of personal decision making and EBP promotes quality nursing care and improves health outcomes for all clients. In addition, for the novice nurse, the process of accessing, applying and evaluating current information within the context of patient need promotes lifelong learning.

9.7 Clinical application of evidence-based practice

Evidence-based practice is now an entrenched element of all aspects of healthcare, practice and delivery. The principles of EBP assist healthcare professionals in identifying knowledge gaps and making informed decisions to complement clinical expertise (Courtney 2005). This text has introduced you to the systematic processes involved in EBP and now it is time to apply the knowledge and skills you have gained.

You now have an opportunity to work through a scenario that may be familiar, as we used it in the case study presented in Chapter 5 (Section 5.5). We have now added more information about the patient, highlighting the complexity you may come across in the clinical area. Using the elements of the EBP process, discuss how you, the clinician, would provide safe and effective care for this patient. You may wish to consider the following key points:

- development of the clinical question/s
- location of the best available evidence and resources to answer the question/s
- critical appraisal of the evidence for its validity and clinical usefulness
- implementation of the evidence and relevant findings into clinical practice, and
- evaluation of outcomes and processes.

CASE STUDY

Mr Allambee is a 50-year-old man of Aboriginal descent with a 5-year history of poorly controlled type 2 diabetes mellitus. He was diagnosed in early 2004 after 2 years of symptoms indicated hyperglycaemia. He is married with two children and is currently self-employed, owning and managing a small grocery store with his wife in the local town shopping centre. One of his daughters works in the family business while studying part-time, while the other lives interstate. He and his wife commute to work each day by car from their property, which is located approximately 1 hour away from the town centre. He has a family history of coronary artery disease. His father died from a heart attack (myocardial infarction) at age 78 and his uncle died at 72 of heart failure several months after suffering a heart attack. Mr Allambee also has the following past medical history:

- hypercholesterolaemia
- inguinal hernia repair 15 years ago
- obstructive sleep apnoea, and
- hypertension.

Upon his initial diagnosis, Mr Allambee was advised to lose weight and cease smoking, but no further action was taken. He previously smoked one packet of cigarettes per day for around 20 years. He now describes himself as a social smoker and social drinker, consuming around three pints of beer during the evening. Furthermore, due to an extremely busy lifestyle, Mr Allambee admits to poor eating habits and an extremely limited exercise regimen. Despite numerous education attempts by his local general practitioner with regards to diabetes self-care management, Mr Allambee admits to not testing his blood glucose levels at home. He currently takes a diverse range of medications, which he suggests he is compliant with 'most of the time'.

Over the past 2 years, Mr Allambee's health has become progressively complicated by his primary diagnosis. He was referred by his general practitioner to a specialist management clinic for increasing foot pain, weight gain and suboptimal diabetes management. Six months ago, Mr Allambee began to experience substernal chest pain and, after a series of investigations, a diagnosis of angina was made. Recently his wife of 20 years has become increasingly concerned because the nature of his chest pain has changed; that is, it occurs on a more frequent basis, lasts longer and develops when he is resting in a chair. She also reports that Mr Allambee frequently complains of nausea, fatigue, shortness of breath and weakness. She states that his medications 'just don't seem to be working anymore'.

A visit to a cardiologist in the city revealed the requirement for a coronary angioplasty. Mr Allambee is worried about the impact his health will have on his family due to his inability to work. He has been admitted to your ward for his angioplasty, and is very worried about his condition.

9.8 **References**

Barredo R 2005 Reflection and evidence-based practice in action: a case based approach. *The Internet Journal of Allied Health Sciences and Practice* 3(3):1–4.

Campbell H, Hotchkiss R, Bradshaw N et al 1998 Integrated care pathways. *British Medical Journal* 316(7125):133–7.

Critical Appraisal Skills Program (CASP) 2009 Critical Appraisal Skills Program (CASP). Available: www.phru.nhs.uk/Pages/PHD/resources.htm 17 May 2009.

Courtney M 2005 *Evidence for nursing practice*. Elsevier, Sydney.

Craig J, Irwig L, Stockler M 2001 Evidence-based medicine: useful tools for decision making. *Medical Journal of Australia* 174(5):248–53.

DiCenso A, Cullum N, Ciliska D 1998 Implementing evidence based nursing: some misconceptions. *Evidence-Based Nursing* 1:38–40.

Dy S M, Garg P, Nyberg D et al 2005 Critical pathway effectiveness: assessing the impact of patient, hospital care and pathway characteristics using qualitative comparative analysis. *Health Services Research* 40(2):499–516.

Every N, Hochman J, Becker R et al 2000 Critical pathways: a review. *Circulation* 101(4):461–5.

Gilbey H J, Ackland T R, Wang A W et al 2003 Exercise improves early functional recovery after total hip arthroplasty. *Clinical Orthopaedics & Related Research* 408:193–200.

Middleton S, Roberts A 2000 *Integrated care pathways: a practical guide to implementation*. Butterworth Heinemann, Edinburgh.

Middleton S, Barnett J, Reeves D 2001 What is an integrated care pathway? *Evidence Based Medicine* 3(3). Available: www.evidence-based-medicine.co.uk 16 May 2009.

Miller M, Kearney N 2004 Guidelines for clinical practice: development, dissemination and implementation. *International Journal of Nursing Studies* 41(7):813–21.

Panella M, Marchisio S, Di Stanislao F 2003 Reducing clinical variations with clinical pathways: do pathways work? *International Journal for Quality in Health Care* 15(6):509–21.

Rooks D S, Huang J, Bierbaum B E et al 2006 Effect of preoperative exercise on measures of functional status in men and women undergoing total hip and knee arthroplasty. *Arthritis & Rheumatism: Arthritis Care & Research* 55(5):700–8.

Sanderlin B, AbdulRahim N 2007 Evidence-based medicine, part 6. An introduction to critical appraisal of clinical practice guidelines. *Journal of the American Osteopathic Association* 7(8):321–4.

Stone P 2002 Popping the (PICO) question in research and evidence-based practice. *Applied Nursing Research* 15(3):197–8.

Thompson C, Cullum N, McCaughan D et al 2004 Nurses, information use, and clinical decision making – the real world potential for evidence-based decisions in nursing. *Evidence-Based Nursing* 7(3):68–72.

Wang A W, Gilbey H J, Ackland T R 2002 Perioperative exercise programs improve early return of ambulatory function after total hip arthroplasty: a randomized, controlled trial. *American Journal of Physical Medicine & Rehabilitation* 81(11):801–6.

Whitney J A, Parkman S 2002 Preoperative physical activity, anesthesia, and analgesia: effects on early postoperative walking after total hip replacement. *Applied Nursing Research* 15(1):19–27.

Whittle C, Hewison A 2007 Integrated care pathways: pathways to change in health care? *Journal of Health Organisation and Management* 21(3):297–306.

Index

Page numbers followed by 'f' denote figures and 't' denote tables.